# Principles of Scientific Literature Evaluation:

# Critiquing Clinical Drug Trials

# Notices

———————————◻———————————

The inclusion in this book of any drug in respect to which patent or trademark rights may exist shall not be deemed, and is not intended as, a grant of or authority to exercise any right or privilege protected by such patent or trademark. All such rights or trademarks are vested in the patent or trademark owner, and no other person may exercise the same without express permission, authority, or license secured from such patent or trademark owner.

The inclusion of a brand name does not mean the author or the publisher has any particular knowledge that the brand listed has properties different from other brands of the same drug, nor should its inclusion be interpreted as an endorsement by the author or publisher. Similarly, the fact that a particular brand has not been included does not indicate the product has been judged to be in any way unsatisfactory or unacceptable. Further, no official support or endorsement of this book by any federal or state agency or pharmaceutical company is intended or inferred.

The nature of drug information is that it is constantly evolving because of ongoing research and clinical experience and is often subject to interpretation. Readers are advised that decisions regarding drug therapy must be based on the independent judgment of the clinician, changing information about a drug (e.g., as reflected in the literature and manufacturers' most current product information), and changing medical practices.

The author and the publisher have made every effort to ensure the accuracy and completeness of the information presented in this book. However, the author and the publisher cannot be held responsible for the continued currency of the information, any inadvertent errors or omissions, or the application of this information.

Therefore, the author and the publisher shall have no liability to any person or entity with regard to claims, loss, or damage caused, or alleged to be caused, directly or indirectly, by the use of information contained herein.

# Principles of Scientific Literature Evaluation:

# Critiquing Clinical Drug Trials

## Frank J. Ascione, Pharm.D., MPH, Ph.D.

Associate Professor of Social and Administrative Sciences and Associate Dean for Academic Affairs

The University of Michigan College of Pharmacy

Ann Arbor, Michigan

American Pharmaceutical Association
Washington, D.C.

Acquiring Editor: Julian I. Graubart
Managing Editor: L. Luan Corrigan
Layout and Graphics: Kathryn A. Stromberger
Cover Designer: Mary Jane Hickey
Proofreader: Kathleen K. Wolter
Indexer: Lillian R. Rodberg

© 2001 by the American Pharmaceutical Association
Published by the American Pharmaceutical Association
2215 Constitution Avenue, N.W.
Washington, DC 20037-2985
www.aphanet.org

To comment on this book via e-mail, send your message to the publisher at
aphabooks@mail.aphanet.org

**Library of Congress Cataloging-in-Publication Data**

Ascione, Frank J., 1946-
    Principles of scientific literature evaluation : critiquing clinical drug trials / Frank J. Ascione
    p.; cm.
    Includes index
    ISBN 1-58212-008-0 (softbound)
      1. Drugs - - Testing - - Evaluation. 2. Clinical trials - - Evaluation. I. Title.

RM301.27 .A834 2001
615'.1'072 - - dc21

                                                                00-045333

How To Order This Book
By phone: 800-878-0729 (802-862-0095 from outside the United States)
VISA®, MasterCard®, and American Express® cards accepted.

# Contents

# Preface

◻

**W**hen I consider using a reference book I usually ask three fundamental questions:

**What does the book contain?**

**Why will it be useful?**

**How should it be used?**

This book represents my experience of more than 30 years as a healthcare practitioner, editor, educator, writer, and researcher. I started thinking about scientific literature evaluation shortly after graduating from pharmacy school in 1969 when I was a practicing hospital pharmacist trying unsuccessfully to find useful drug information to give patients and physicians.

My interest continued when I received my Doctor of Pharmacy degree in 1973 and moved to Washington, D.C. to participate in the American Pharmaceutical Association's Drug Interactions Evaluation Program, which was responsible for producing the publication *Evaluations of Drug Interactions*. When reviewing the scientific literature about well-known drug interactions, I was surprised to find how little clinical evidence existed to document relatively well-known interactions. Based on this experience, I became interested in educating healthcare providers about how to better use drug information sources.

This interest in teaching was fulfilled when I returned to the University of Michigan in 1976 to study for a Ph.D. and began teaching a course at the College of Pharmacy on drug information and scientific literature evaluation in 1977. I continue to teach that course today and have introduced hundreds of pharmacy students to the critical reading skills necessary to understand and evaluate the scientific literature about drug therapy. I first published my approach to scientific literature evaluation as part of the 1994 reference book *Principles of Drug Information and Scientific Literature Evaluation*. The current textbook is an expanded and revised version of the 1994 reference.

The current book is useful because it is intended to aid the healthcare practitioner in understanding the scientific and regulatory basis of drug information and scientific literature evaluation. The increased complexity of drug therapy, coupled with the continual demand to effectively manage the direct costs of drugs, has necessitated that healthcare practitioners make difficult decisions regarding what drugs to use and how to use them. These difficult decisions require a fundamental understanding of the evidence about the drug's effectiveness and safety.

How to use this book? The book is flexible enough to accommodate the needs of the less experienced student as well as the more experienced but busy healthcare practitioner. Perhaps the best way to use the book is to follow the stepwise approach outlined within. This approach consists of a series of questions about different aspects of articles describing clinical drug trials. The questions were developed from the numerous guidelines published by other authors and modified by me during the many years teaching this subject matter to students. In my class, I review each question in the order in which it is presented in the book. This method allows the user to systematically obtain the information needed to critically read the scientific literature.

Instead of using the stepwise approach, the reader can also obtain specific information about certain aspects of an article or a clinical drug trial by simply going to the comprehensive index and finding the appropriate section. Each question or section is written to be inclusive, with cross references to other sections of the book where appropriate. For those readers who wish to learn more than the information provided in the book, an extensive list of references is provided, and all statements are thoroughly documented.

I often tell my students at the beginning of my course that they will read the scientific literature differently after they complete the course. I hope that everyone who reads this book will have the same experience.

Frank J. Ascione
December 2000

# Acknowledgments

—————————————◻—————————————

*This book is dedicated to Gloria Francke, whose confidence in my abilities made my preparation of this material possible.*

*Many others also contributed to this effort. Thanks to Patty, Wendy, and Mark for their lifelong support. Thanks also to my previous co-authors, Carol Manifold and Mary Parenti, for giving me the insight that allowed me to be the sole author of this current version. I am also grateful to Rivka Siden, who provided me with valuable assistance and wisdom during the teaching of my course on scientific literature evaluation.*

*Friends and colleagues such as J&J, Ira Cohen, and Duane Kirking provided assistance throughout the past years and that has been greatly appreciated. Thanks to Julian Graubart of APhA for his patience and guidance in getting this book published. My gratitude also is given to L. Luan Corrigan, who edited this book for APhA and who has been my friend, professional colleague, and editorial instructor since 1973.*

*Special thanks to Nancy Cunningham, who provided valuable editorial assistance and support during the initial preparation of this book.*

# 1  Evaluating the Scientific Literature

Most prescription drug product information is generated as manufacturers attempt to develop products for which a potentially large market exists. (A possible exception is orphan drugs, i.e., drugs targeted for relatively small patient populations for which the government subsidizes research.) Another primary source of information is the federal government, which sponsors the development of drugs through entities such as the National Cancer Institute.[1]

Drug product information is provided to a variety of constituents, although two have been traditionally considered the most important. One audience is the Food and Drug Administration (FDA), which is responsible for the regulation of drug development through the drug approval and marketing process. Another audience is the clinical community that includes physicians, pharmacists, and nurses. These individuals are responsible for the proper use of medications in the clinical setting.[2, 3]

While providing relevant information to the FDA and the clinical community is a major focus of pharmaceutical manufacturers, other groups are emerging, such as healthcare institutions and managed care organizations, which are responsible for ensuring that medications are used in a cost–benefit manner. Another emerging group is the patient and the general public, who are gaining greater influence on medication use through

- the switch of a significant number of medications from prescription to nonprescription status,

- the extensive use of direct-to-consumer advertising, and

- greater political advocacy for diseases such as AIDS and Alzheimer's disease.

Members of the investment community, whose primary goal is to maximize return on investment, are an important but less public audience.[3]

Manufacturer-generated information is comprehensive but tends to focus only on what is needed to get a drug product approved and used in clinical practice. Thus, gaps in knowledge about the drug exist; such gaps are often addressed by other groups. One such group is the federal government, which funds basic and applied drug research. An example is the Pediatric Pharmacology Research Unit of the National Institute of Child Health and Human Development. This unit was established to address the traditional problem of the lack of drug testing in children, which resulted in an inadequate information base for using drugs in children.[4]

Another example is the Surrogate Marker Collaborative Group (SMCG), formed in 1996. This group consists of representatives from industry, academia, and governmental science and research agencies. This group examines the value of surrogate markers (indirect measures of outcomes) in predicting the value of HIV therapies and shares data that provide insight into this value. Other sources of information are healthcare institutions, which focus on generating drug data about the effective use of the drug product after it has entered the United States healthcare market.[5–7]

The result of this multiple effort is an explosion of diverse and sometimes contradictory information. Unfortunately, the growth is also accompanied by variations in research quality. While many clinical drug trials are methodologically sound, biases may exist in the overall publication process. The primary bias is the tendency to report only "positive" results and not findings that are "negative." Other biases result from the pressure on scientists to publish, causing some to engage in misleading practices such as

- making exaggerated claims for their findings,

- fragmenting their results by reporting in multiple journals,

- conducting and submitting for publication only those clinical drug trials that can be completed and published easily, or

- providing incomplete descriptions of trial methods and/or results.

A more serious problem which, fortunately, occurs rarely, is scientific fraud, where false data are created or conflicting or undesirable results are withheld (*see* Chapter 2, Questions 2 and 3).[8–19]

Thus, the healthcare practitioner is forced to decide which set of conflicting or contradictory findings is most representative of typical clinical practice, even though all of the research examined may be considered methodologically sound (*see* Chapter 9, Question 23). The need to choose among conflicting or incomplete results may confuse healthcare practitioners about optimal drug therapy.[5,8,20–26]

The multitude of drug information sources has changed the approach that healthcare practitioners should use for clinical practice and education. The traditional approach was knowledge disseminated from experts and interpreted by the perspective and experience of the individual healthcare practitioner. The new approach is based on the review of multiple sources of information and focuses on a comprehensive assessment of the quality of the information provided. This approach is commonly referred to as "evidenced-based medicine." The practice of evidence-based medicine means integrating individual expertise with the best external evidence from systematic research.[5,27]

The evidence-based approach focuses on identifying key issues within the decision-making process and locating the "best" evidence that is both valid and applicable, estimating the benefits and harm to patients, and identifying gaps in the science. An understanding of that evidence requires a familiarity with the scientific literature that supports it.[5,27]

This chapter provides an overview of the type of drug information available to the public, including how and why it is generated. A primary focus is on the scientific and regulatory basis of the drug approval process used in the United States. Information is also provided on research designs to evaluate drug therapy and the scientific rationale for their use. Finally, a structured approach to evaluating the quality of published articles is described.

## Drug Approval Process

A key to understanding how drug information is generated is to understand the drug approval process in the United States. In this country, manufacturers have generally assumed responsibility for identifying, developing, and testing new drugs. This development program turns promising chemicals into useful drug products. Specifically, this process focuses on "identifying the right drug for specific indications and determining the appropriate regimen of administration." The process requires scientific expertise from different disciplines and an enormous amount of time and money. The testing begins with animals to determine whether the drug candidate has a pharmacological property that may successfully alter a human disease process and that it does not have a toxicity profile that could cause adverse events if given in therapeutically effective doses.[3,28-30]

The FDA closely monitors this complex and expensive process, primarily through its Center for Drug Evaluation and Research (CDER). The center's major responsibility is to evaluate the benefits and risks associated with new drug products before they can be marketed. CDER is part of the United States' oldest consumer protection agency and is currently the largest of the FDA's centers. The FDA usually becomes involved when a drug shows clinical promise.[31]

The FDA's (and CDER's) regulatory responsibility has evolved since the beginning of the 20th century. This evolution can be divided into phases:

- Ensuring drug purity.
- Assuring drug safety.

■ Promoting drug efficacy.

■ Encouraging the development of drugs.

The first phase, ensuring drug purity, started with the passage of the Biologics Control Act of 1902, which required the licensing of serums and vaccines. Four years later, in 1906, the first major attempt to control drug quality occurred with the Federal Food and Drug Act. This act required that drugs meet standards of strength and purity, although the burden of proof was on the FDA.[32-35]

The second phase, assuring drug safety, began with the revamping of federal regulations after deaths were reported due to a poisonous substance in a liquid product containing sulfanilamide. In 1938, the Food, Drug, and Cosmetic Act (FDCA) was passed; it mandated pre-market FDA safety review of new drug products.[32-35]

The third phase, promoting drug efficacy, began with the Kefauver–Harris amendments to the FDCA. These amendments were in response to concerns about the regulation of drug availability generated by thousands of birth malformations caused by thalidomide, a popular drug used in Europe. The drug was never approved for use in the United States, but the public wanted to strengthen protection. Thus, the amendments required that drugs be both safe and effective before they were marketed, and the burden of proof was on the manufacturer. An important result was that manufacturers were required to conduct sophisticated and well-designed clinical trials to demonstrate efficacy and safety. In addition, the drug manufacturer was required to send data about adverse drug events (ADEs) to the FDA and to provide complete product information to physicians.[32-35]

The current phase, encouraging drug development, began in response to public criticisms about the FDA being overly protective in approving drugs. Critics argued that a "drug lag" existed in the United States: compared to other industrialized countries, fewer new drugs were approved and the length of time for approval was much longer. Several legislative steps were taken to improve and accelerate the drug approval process.[36-38]

The first prominent legislation in this phase was the Orphan Drug Act of 1983, by which manufacturers were encouraged to develop drug products for treating rare diseases. Because of the small number of patients affected, there was little or no financial incentive for manufacturers to develop drugs to treat such diseases. The act offered tax deductions and patent extensions. Other prominent attempts to promote the availability of drug products were the Drug Price Competition and Patent Term Restoration Act of 1984 and the FDA Modernization Act of 1997, which promotes a speedier FDA approval process, especially for drugs to treat life-threatening diseases such as AIDS. [6,39,40]

## Looking at the Process

The drug approval process begins when a drug sponsor, usually a pharmaceutical company, seeks to develop a new drug with a potential for a useful and profitable place in the market. The process has distinct stages with different objectives (Table 1-1). The first is the drug discovery and development stage, in which the pharmacology of a chemical compound is explored in appropriate animal models to determine whether the compound, or class of compounds, alters a disease process and thus has potential human therapeutic benefit. The type of research performed in this stage includes preliminary studies to determine the chemical's (or class of chemicals') potential and is focused on understanding the toxicity of the drug (at very high doses), its potential pharmacokinetic and pharmacodynamic profile, and type of formulation needed for human use.[30,41]

The preclinical development stage is next, and here the research focuses primarily on collecting evidence that the drug could be tested safely in humans. Studies involve determining toxicity under acute or short-term conditions. Additional information about pharmacokinetics and metabolism is collected from animal models. Some research may also be conducted during this stage to determine the best route and frequency of administration, outline the drug's mechanism of action, and further explore the drug candidate's pharmacology profile to see if it might be useful for other diseases.[30]

The role of the FDA in the early stages of drug research is small, partially because of regulatory restrictions. The Food, Drug, and Cosmetic Act requires the FDA to ensure that the new drugs developed are safe and effective but does not give the agency responsibility for developing new drugs. FDA involvement in the drug development process occurs when the preclinical research sponsored by the manufacturer indicates that the drug has potential clinical benefits in humans. Once the evidence is presented to the FDA, agency staff and a local institutional review board review the sponsor's plan for clinical testing in humans. The clinical testing phase begins once the protocol has been approved.[41,42]

The clinical testing part of drug development is divided into four stages that are typically called phase I, II, III, and IV research which will be discussed more comprehensively in the next section. Although the objectives of each phase are different, the phases are not entirely separate entities because the information obtained from one phase provides the basis for the next. From a regulatory and scientific perspective, it is imperative that stringent scientific methodology is used throughout these stages to minimize the effect of coincidence, poor design, and research bias on the analysis of the results.[43]

Phase I and II clinical trials involve the initial human experiments to define the investigational drug's safety, tolerance, and pharmacokinetics in normal volunteers and the drug's initial efficacy

**Table 1-1** Drug Discovery, Development, and Approval Process [30, 33, 41]

| Stage | Description | Duration |
|---|---|---|
| **Discovery and product development** | Synthesis of chemical compounds to identify those with potential for biologic activity. Use of in vitro and in vivo animal studies to examine potential pharmacology of chemical. | 1–3 years |
| **Pre-clinical** | More comprehensive testing of drug product stability, formulation development, validation of biologic activity, examination of toxicity, pharmacokinetics, and mechanism of action (pharmacodynamics). Testing done in vitro and in animals. | 1–5 years |
| **Clinical trials: phase I** | Focus on drug safety and tolerance. Objective is to determine safe dosing levels, pharmacokinetic profile, and preferred route of administration. Performed on 20–100 healthy volunteers or special populations. | 1 week to 1 month |
| **Clinical trials: phase II** | Determination of safe and effective dose range, evaluations of pharmacokinetics following a multiple-dose schedule, establishment and validation of biochemical marker levels in humans, and identification of metabolic pathway. Drug is tested on 100–400 patients who represent the intended population, usually without serious concomitant illnesses. | Several months to 2 years |
| **Clinical trials: phase III** | Conducting randomized, double-blind, controlled studies on a wide range of patients representing the target population, and small-scale pharmacokinetic studies in special populations such as pediatric age groups or renal- or hepatic-impaired patients. Purpose is to establish safety and effectiveness in a varied, large population of patients over an extended time period. Testing is performed on several hundred to several thousand patients. | Several months to several (usually no more than 4) years |
| **Clinical trials: phase IV** | Also known as postmarketing surveillance studies. Focus is to provide additional data on drug safety and to confirm the clinical benefit of the drug, including expanding the indications for its use. May involve small number (50) to several thousand patients. | Several months to years with safety surveillance throughout product life. |

in patients. In addition, the nonclinical research program is continued to learn more about the drug's mechanism of action. Phase III clinical studies involve more intensive research on a more diverse set of patients. The objective is to collect more safety information and to confirm the investigational drug's clinical efficacy. Where appropriate, human pharmacokinetic studies evaluate potential changes in the drug's characteristics caused by age, sex, race, interaction with other drugs, disease state, and hepatic and renal dysfunction. While the clinical research in this phase is centered on efficacy and safety, animal research continues and focuses on learning more about the investigational drug's carcinogenicity, its effects on the fetus, and its pharmacokinetic profile.[30]

Once a drug has been approved, the sponsor begins distribution of the drug product and its promotion to physicians, pharmacists, patients, and other appropriate decision-makers. Some of this promotion is based on additional information gained from phase IV clinical drug research, especially in the area of drug safety (commonly referred to as postmarketing surveillance).[3]

The postmarketing surveillance phase requires manufacturers to monitor the known effects discovered during the drug approval process as well as any additional effects identified after release. Once a product is marketed, there are many more patients exposed to the drug, including those with multiple medical problems undergoing treatment with other drugs (*see* Chapter 5, Question 14).[3]

## Specific Stages

It is estimated that for every 1000 compounds screened for pharmacological activity in animals, only 100 have the necessary biological activity and safety profile for evaluation in humans. If all 100 drugs were submitted to the FDA for clinical testing via a new drug application (and they are not), about 70% would successfully complete phase I and go on to phase II; 33% of the original 100 would complete phase 2 and go to phase III, and 25–30% would clear phase III (and, on average, about 20 of the original 100 would ultimately be approved for marketing). The low success rate is due to many factors; the primary reason is that results from animal models are poorly correlated with biological activity and/or safety in humans.[30,42,44]

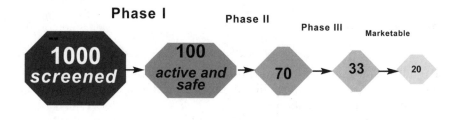

The clinical research performed during development is complex and shaped by the information required for the new drug application (NDA). The research can be divided into two distinct stages: clinical trials needed for market approval and postapproval trials required to ensure safe and effective use of the drug once it is released to the marketplace (Table 1-1).

## Premarketing Clinical Drug Trials

The clinical research required for drug approval by the FDA usually lasts from two years (for fast-track drugs indicated for the treatment of life-threatening diseases such as AIDS) up to 10 years. From a regulatory perspective, the research is divided into phase I, II, and III trials and may involve thousands of patients and subjects before it is completed.

### Phase I clinical trials

Phase I clinical trials[33,42,45] represent the first use of the drug in humans and is the shortest phase. The objectives are to determine

- the organs most adversely affected by various dosing levels,
- a pharmacokinetic and pharmacodynamic profile, and
- a preferred route of administration.

The trials involve various doses and schedules to focus on initial drug safety and pharmacokinetics.

Phase I studies usually involve only a small number of subjects, from 20 to 100 normal healthy adult volunteers, divided into small treatment groups, generally about 10 per group. The actual trial design varies with the type of drug evaluated, but most studies are single-dose trials. However, multiple-dose trials may be used for short time periods. In special cases, where the drug has known toxicity, it may be given to subjects who have the disease or condition for which the drug is indicated.[33,42,45]

Most phase I clinical trials last no more than a month, although some continue for several months. If evidence from phase I clinical trials suggests that the drug may not be safe for human use, its development is stopped. Seventy percent of phase I drugs progress to the next stage. [33,42,45]

### Phase II clinical trials

Phase II clinical trials[33,42,45,46] represent the introduction of the new drug into the intended population to demonstrate the drug's effectiveness and learn more about the drug's safety. For the first time, information is collected about

- the drug's minimum effective dose,
- the dose range for clinical efficacy,
- the drug's efficacy in varying stages of the disease, and
- the magnitude and duration of the effect.

Additional information is collected about the drug's safety, pharmacokinetic/pharmacodynamic profile, and biochemical/metabolic pathway.

The research in this phase usually consists of controlled pilot studies on a limited number (100–400) of patients who usually are not suffering from other serious illnesses or taking concurrent medications. Patients are typically randomized to a treatment group taking the drug or a control group taking a placebo. In cases where a placebo drug would be unethical, such as in cancer patients, a comparative drug is administered to the patients in the control group. The trial typically lasts from several months to two years.[33,42,45]

Phase II clinical trials address two fundamental questions for the manufacturer:

*Is the drug effective in the dose range established by the sponsor?*

*Is the potential effectiveness likely to make an impact on the drug market?*

A company decides if the cost of further research (in phase III and IV trials) and subsequent marketing efforts are worthwhile. Thus, this phase is critical in development because it provides clinical information at a low cost to determine whether substantial future financial investment is desirable.[46]

### Phase III clinical trials

The decision to embark on phase III studies[33,42,45] is critical. Drug development from preclinical research through phase II trials is relatively inexpensive compared to phase III research. The number and size of the studies increase dramatically. Phase III research

- establishes safety and effectiveness in a varied, large population of patients over an extended time period,
- collects additional information on the drug's safety profile, particularly the incidence and type of side effects that occur during an extended time, and
- collects information relative to
  the frequency of rare side effects,
  drug–drug interactions,
  relative toxicity compared to drugs already marketed,

drug administration characteristics (e.g., the preferred
dosage form),
the drug's half-life in impaired populations, and
the overall pharmacokinetic/pharmacodynamic profile.

In some cases, information about the drug's relative value compared to other agents currently on the market is collected, specifically its comparative efficacy and safety profile (*see* Chapter 5, Question 14).

Phase III clinical trials expand evaluation to larger numbers of patients (several hundred to several thousand, generally not exceeding 3000 patients) for substantially longer time periods (months to several years, usually not more than 4 years.). The investigational drug is generally compared to a placebo to establish clinical efficacy, although it may be compared to the currently accepted standard treatment of the disease under study. The research is rigorous and includes randomized, double-blind, controlled studies on a wide range of patients representing the target population. Small-scale pharmacokinetic studies in special populations such children or renal- or hepatic-impaired patients may also be done.[33,42,45]

Phase III trials are the longest, most expensive, and most complex aspect of the clinical drug research process and require careful monitoring by the drug sponsor and the FDA. At the completion of phase III research, the FDA's decision to approve a drug for marketing is based on evidence that the drug provides substantial clinical benefit and is safe to use under normal conditions. When the review is complete, the FDA indicates if the drug

- is approved,

- is approvable provided minor changes are made, or

- is not approved because of major problems.

In the last case, the applicant amends or withdraws the NDA or asks for a hearing. The drug can be marketed after FDA approval when the drug sponsor gets its production and distribution systems operational.[34]

## Postapproval Trials

Clinical research does not end when a drug is approved to be marketed. In fact, clinical research in the postmarketing phase continues throughout the market life of the drug product. This type of research is traditionally referred to as phase IV clinical research. The term "phase IV" is fairly standard and covers the vast majority of postmarketing clinical research about a drug. Phase IV trials are also referred to as "marketing studies," "experience studies," or "drug effectiveness studies" to emphasize that they are conducted after the drug is marketed, rather than prior to its approval. Other terms such as "seeding trials" or "observational studies" are inappropriate because they generally refer to efforts made by marketing departments to encourage physicians to prescribe the new drug. Phase IV trials are commonly also referred to as postmarketing surveillance, although some experts believe the latter term primarily refers to the process of monitoring the safety of a marketed drug.[33,47,48]

Information typically gathered in phase IV clinical trials includes

- the proper dosing for specific groups such as the elderly,

- limitations of use in patients with certain pathologies such as renal or hepatic impairment, and

- the existence and incidence of less frequent, but important, side effects.

Although the type of research in phase IV varies depending on the needs of the various constituents, it may involve trials similar to those in phase III, ADE monitoring (sometimes called pharmacovigilance), long-term epidemiological trials (generally called pharmacoepidemiology), pooled interpretation of multiple small-scale trials (meta-analyses), or cost–effectiveness research (usually labeled as pharmacoeconomics). The research ranges from a single patient to several thousand. The duration of these studies is variable, lasting several months to several years, although safety surveillance continues throughout the product lifetime.

Phase IV trials require the same level of monitoring and quality assurance as phase III trials and often generate results published in scientific journals. Thus, the data are viewed not only by regulatory agencies but also by other interested readers such as members of the health-care professions, the medical press, and, more recently, the general public.[33,47–49]

### Purpose

Phase IV clinical research demonstrates[3,33,48] the value of the drug to patients and healthcare practitioners and administrators (*see* Chapter 5, Question 14). Another purpose is to extend knowledge about the drug's efficacy and safety. The drug sponsor may need to know more about the drug product for marketing or product liability purposes, further regulatory requirements of the FDA, or the market needs of various constituents such as healthcare organizations.

Information about drug costs and long-term effects is also desirable. A specific regulatory requirement that the drug sponsor must follow is the continual monitoring of the drug's safety through structured postmarketing surveillance. Also studied are additional therapeutic effects identified subsequent to the release of the marketed drug.[33,48]

The results of these efforts have both positive and negative consequences for the drug sponsor. A positive effect might expand product use through the identification of new uses (often called "off label indications"). Another positive outcome would be a better understanding of how to use the drug safely. The most significant negative consequence is the discovery that the drug is more hazardous than originally anticipated. The result may be a labeling change or, in more serious cases, removal of the drug from the market by the FDA, which has the regulatory authority if such action is deemed appropriate. Removal from the market often occurs because the FDA lacks authority to limit distribution or use (although it has successfully done so with certain drug products).[3,33,48]

### Differences from other forms of clinical research

Phase III clinical trials performed for regulatory purposes usually include a relatively narrow range of patients, and the results obtained are not all generalizable to the population at large (*see* Chapter 3, Question 8, and Chapter 9, Question 23). Phase IV clinical studies, in contrast, include a broader patient sample that more closely reflects medical practice. These populations may include patients excluded during the premarketing research such as children, women of childbearing age, and the elderly. Because phase I–III trials should demonstrate that the drug has biological activity and clinical efficacy, patients receiving the investigational drug are often compared with patients receiving a placebo or no drug treatment (*see* Chapter 4, Question 11).[5,33,47,49–51]

Phase IV trials assess the relative merit of a newly marketed drug compared to other available treatments. Phase IV studies also focus on hypotheses and questions that could not be addressed in premarketing trials due to the small number of patients and limited time, such as the possibility of long-term toxicity.[4,33,47,49–51]

The differences between postmarketing phase IV trials and premarketing phase I–III trials are not always clear, especially the comparison of phase III and phase IV research. Many patient advocate groups sponsor comparative clinical drug studies in cardiovascular disease, cancer, or AIDS and call them phase III trials, regardless of regulatory approval. Patients with serious, life-threatening diseases such as AIDS or advanced cancer may get a product prior to its approval through "expanded access," "compassionate need," or "treatment IND" programs designed to speed up drug approval by providing products to patients more quickly. Such studies, even though they take place before drug approval, share characteristics with phase IV trials.[5,40,47–53]

For life-threatening diseases, new drugs may also go through an "accelerated approval" process in which the new drug is marketed based on limited data and under the condition that further evidence will be provided from well-controlled trials completed later. These subsequent studies, even though they take place after new drug approval, share many characteristics with phase III clinical trials.[4,40,47-53]

### Drug safety

The FDA collects safety data[47,54-57] throughout the drug approval process. In the premarketing phase, the FDA maintains a database consisting of both animal and human data. The animal data are important to the agency when decisions are made regarding the safety of proceeding from preclinical research to phase I-III research. Besides establishing overall drug safety, animal data help establish dose require-ments and the administration schedule for the initial stages of clinical research (phase I clinical trials). The animal data complement human data in areas where insufficient information may exist about drug safety such as the carcinogenicity or teratogenicity of a particular agent. Premarketing safety assessment must be established in two ways. First, the drug sponsor must demonstrate that all reasonable testing occurred regarding drug safety. Second, based on those tests, the drug must be reasonably safe for its proposed indication.

The premarketing database is insufficient for assessing a drug's overall safety, primarily because of insufficient numbers of patients. Most premarketing drug development (phase I-III trials) involves about 3000 patients, but this sample is not large or representative enough to detect rare events that may occur in less than 1% of the patients. A second limitation is the duration of drug exposure. Although premarket research may take up to 10 years, individual drug trials are generally shorter than a year. Even trials of investigational drugs intended for chronic administration are limited to several years and may be insufficient to duplicate the longer periods of use.

A third limitation is theoretical. The clinical drug development program tests a hypothesis about a drug's efficacy, with the assumption (based on animal data and phase I and II trials) that the drug is reasonably safe. Although phase III trials are large enough to detect true differences between the experimental drug and a control drug or placebo, the theoretical approach to detecting ADEs is different because such effects are, by definition, infrequent and unexpected events. Thus, the endpoints to study are usually not known, which makes assessing drug safety difficult.[47,54-57]

The agency approach to overcoming these limitations is to estimate the potential risks for the drug and to pool the data to increase the likelihood that differences in the toxicity profile of the experimental drug can be identified compared to the controls (*see* Chapter 5, Question 14).

While the premarketing assessment of drug risk is rigorous and conservative, it is still limited compared to postmarketing surveillance. Phase I–III trials usually identify the common adverse events and possibly some serious but less frequent adverse reactions. These trials also may identify areas where additional toxic reactions may occur, such as in the liver.[57]

Nevertheless, it is not uncommon for a drug, once approved and in use, to be used at higher doses and for longer duration than in the premarketing trials. In addition, patients in the postmarketing clinical setting tend to be more heterogeneous in terms of the presence of multiple diseases and the use of concurrent medications compared to the relatively "pure" premarketing subjects.[57]

Phase I–III clinical trials provide preliminary evidence, rather than proof, of the safety of a drug; phase IV trials are needed to provide additional documentation. If properly controlled and closely monitored, such trials yield a more reliable safety profile than any method of spontaneous reporting of ADEs, such as yellow cards, case reports, literature screening, and so forth. In particular, the number of patients exposed to the drug is better known in a prospective trial and, therefore, the true incidence of ADEs can be estimated accurately.[47]

Phase IV clinical trials are relatively effective in identifying rare and unpredictable ADEs. While common ADEs are well documented by the time the investigational drug is marketed, rare ADEs require the treatment of a larger number of patients to be detected. Large numbers of patients are rarely available at the time of granting marketing authorization to a new drug, and seldom even after early phase IV trials. This lack justifies long-term surveillance monitoring for drug safety.[47]

## Interpreting Different Drug Research Designs

The information about drugs is commonly categorized as "primary," "secondary," and "tertiary" sources.[58]

**Primary sources:** usually articles about original research or case reports; provide significant detail and new knowledge about drugs.

**Secondary sources:** indexing or abstracting services such as Medline; generally used to locate primary drug literature.

**Tertiary sources:** resources such as textbooks that provide an overview of the drug topic; generally do not contain as much detail as primary or secondary resources.

The focus of this book is on primary literature sources. Such sources contain information on research designs used in the drug development and use process. To interpret the reported results for clinical practice, the healthcare practitioner needs to be familiar with the advantages and disadvantages of each design. The typical designs used are animal studies, case-control or cohort studies, pharmacoeconomic studies, anecdotal or spontaneous reporting, N of 1 studies, meta-analysis, and clinical drug trials.

## Animal Studies

Drug research in animals[30,44,59] generally focuses on the drug's pharmacodynamic and pharmacokinetic profiles. In addition, animal models are used to predict the level and incidence of the drug's toxicity. Animal studies are commonly done in the preclinical phase of drug development but continue concurrently when the clinical research phase begins to refine the drug's dosing parameters and safety profile.

The results of animal research should be applied cautiously in the clinical setting because effects observed in humans may not be manifested in animals and vice versa. Use of animal models to predict drug effects in humans may lead to erroneous projections because of species differences in the rate and degree of drug absorption, distribution, metabolism, and excretion.[30,44,59]

## Case-Control or Cohort Studies

Case-control or cohort studies[47,48,57,60–63] are often used in phase IV clinical trials and are sometimes called pharmacoepidemiology, drug utilization review, or postmarketing surveillance. These studies tend to be performed on large, diverse populations and to focus on general use of the drug. Case-control or retrospective studies go back in time to determine what characteristics are associated with a particular drug effect. Thus, patients with a certain disease or set of symptoms (which could be an ADE) are examined to determine whether they were taking the drug under research.

An example of a case-control study is a clinical drug trial that examined the effect of antidepressants on the risk of falls by nursing home residents. By using a patient database that consisted of residents of nursing homes in Tennessee, the investigators identified 2428 patients who were new users of three types of antidepressants: tricyclic antidepressants (665 subjects), selective serotonin-reuptake inhibitors (612 subjects), trazodone (304 subjects), or nonusers of antidepressants (847 subjects) during a time period selected retrospectively by the investigators. The incidence of falls reported in the database for each group during the time period selected was compared. The results indicated that the users of antidepressants had higher rates of falls than nonusers but that no significant differences occurred among the different antidepressants.[61]

Cohort or prospective studies differ from case-control studies because they typically begin with patients taking the drug under research and follow the patients for an extended time to determine if they develop any ADEs. An example is the prospective study that examined the value of folic acid in the prevention of birth defects in pregnant women. In this study, 4753 pregnant women were randomly assigned to receive a multivitamin supplement that included folic acid or a supplement that included trace elements and vitamin C but no folic acid. The women were followed throughout their pregnancies, and information about the births of their children was collected and compared. The results showed a lower overall incidence of birth defects in the group receiving the multivitamin supplement compared to the women receiving the trace element, particularly in the incidence of neural tube defects.[63]

Case-control and cohort studies are good techniques for assessing the hazards of drug use in clinical practice, and the results tend to be generalizable because the conditions are similar. However, causal relationships are more difficult to establish with this type of design compared with clinical drug trials. This difficulty is generally due to the inability to accurately determine the timing of the drug administration in relation to the clinical outcome and the failure to control for the influence of other possible causative factors[60–62] (*see* Chapter 9, Question 22).

## Pharmacoeconomic Studies

Pharmacoeconomic research[64–66] has received a great deal of attention recently because of the need to manage healthcare costs. Its focus is to identify, measure, and compare the costs (i.e., resources consumed) and consequences of pharmaceutical products and services (*see* Chapter 5, Question 14). Pharmacoeconomic research is done infrequently in the premarketing stage but is often performed after the approval to help market the product. Unfortunately, the rush to conduct pharmacoeconomic studies has resulted in wide variation in quality and rigor and the rampant misuse of terms such as "cost-effectiveness." Formulas used to measure costs vary widely and produce significantly different results. Nevertheless, pharmacoeconomic research is useful in providing additional information about the potential impact of a drug's clinical use.

## Anecdotal or Spontaneous Reporting

Anecdotal or spontaneous reports[44,67–69] (sometimes called case reports) are often used in phase IV research to identify unexpected, infrequent, or previously undetected ADEs. The drug manufacturer is required to collect such reports and provide them to the FDA, if necessary. Spontaneous reports are also collected by the FDA's MedWatch program. In this program, healthcare practitioners are encouraged to submit information to the FDA regarding serious ADEs. This information is important for monitoring drug safety and can lead to significant changes in the manufacturer's product labeling. It also sometimes results in the removal of a drug from the marketplace, such as the decision to withdraw the antihypertensive drug mibefradil after serious ADEs were reported.[44]

Although clinical drug trials have generally replaced case reports as the source of information about drug efficacy, case reports can be useful when decisions cannot be made based on controlled trials. An example would be an unexpected side effect that could be ultimately redefined as a therapeutic effect if certain dosing and drug monitoring conditions are changed. The value of case reports for identifying drug effectiveness is enhanced if two or more treatments are present, repeated measures are implemented, and appropriate statistical analysis techniques are used to determine the significance of the reported data.[67,68]

Despite their value, case reports do not replace clinical drug trials as the main source of data regarding the benefits and hazards of drug therapy. Their disadvantages include the lack of information to establish a causal relationship between the drug and the reported outcome, underreporting of events (especially ADEs), and biases due to observations made under uncontrolled conditions.[69]

## N of 1 Studies

A derivation of the case report is a research scheme in which a single patient is exposed to both the investigational drug and a placebo or an alternative treatment (which is usually assigned randomly). The method is usually referred to as a "N of 1 study" but has also been labeled a "single case experiment" or "intensive research design." N of 1 studies[67,68] are different from case reports and other controlled designs (*see* Chapter 4, Question 10) because the focus is on assessing the benefit of drug treatment for an individual patient, not the overall effect on a group of patients. The primary purpose of N of 1 studies is to find the best treatment for a particular patient. Therefore, the results of N of 1 studies should be applied to only the patients who participate in the study. However, the designs are more advantageous than case reports because the patient is given the drug under controlled conditions.[67,68]

## Meta-Analysis

Meta-analysis[70–75] is a statistical analysis that combines the results from different clinical drug trials to arrive at a single conclusion about an investigational drug. Meta-analysis involves several steps. The published literature about a drug treatment is collected and reviewed. Only those clinical drug trials that meet a set of design criteria are selected. The data are then pooled, and the "effect size" is calculated. The effect size is the estimation of the pooled difference between the investigational drug and the various control treatments. The pooled difference can be the average difference between experimental and control groups or a weighted difference that rewards better designed studies. The statistical significance and the clinical importance of the differences are then evaluated.

Meta-analysis is a useful technique because of its value in identifying previously undetected drug effects by pooling data to create a larger sample of patients. However, meta-analysis is not as useful if the clinical drug trials analyzed are poorly designed or if a significant number of trials have different outcome measures.[70–75]

## Clinical Drug Trials

Pocock[76] defines the clinical drug trial as "any form of planned experiment that involves patients and is designed to elucidate the most appropriate treatment of future patients with a given medical condition." Clinical drug trials[42,43,77,78] are considered to be the most effective tool for the evaluation of drug therapy and are the main topic of the remainder of this book.

# Evaluation of Clinical Drug Trials

Although clinical drug trials have contributed greatly to the effective and safe use of drugs, there are difficulties with the interpretation, feasibility, and ethics of these trials. Because some difficulties are due to a lack of adequate understanding of the purpose and design of clinical drug trials, Chapters 2–9 discuss how to understand and apply this type of research. These chapters are organized by the typical sections of a published article (Table 1-2).[42,43,77–79]

**Table 1-2** Typical Structure of Articles Describing Clinical Drug Trials [76,80]

| Section | Description |
|---------|-------------|
| **Title** | Brief description of the research conducted |
| **Abstract** | Overview of the research conducted |
| **Introduction** | Background information for the trials, including results of prior research |
| **Methods** | Description of drug research design (e.g., criteria for subject selection and number, dosing information, experimental and control groups, measures of efficacy and safety) |
| **Results** | Analysis of research findings, including discussion of dropouts, discontinuation of drug therapy |
| **Discussion/ Conclusions** | Interpretation of results, comparison to current standard drug treatment, discussion of future implications of research |
| **References** | Evidence that prior research has been considered in designing and interpreting the trials |

The consistent structure of the articles enables the healthcare practitioner to identify important aspects of the trial relatively easily. Nevertheless, an organized approach is needed to identify the comparatively few papers that are most applicable to clinical practice. Many schemes are available that address how a healthcare practitioner should evaluate the results generated from clinical drug trials. The evaluation process discussed in this book is a hybrid of most of those efforts and is described comprehensively in Chapters 2 through 9. The checklist on the next page shows an overview of the evaluation scheme. Whenever possible, examples of various clinical drug trials are provided to assist in comprehending the principles discussed.[60,79–83]

## Abstract and Introduction

☐ 1. How clear and complete are the trial title and abstract?
☐ 2. Is the article in a journal using a comprehensive review system to ensure quality?
☐ 3. Are there important sources of biases in the author(s)' background or funding source?
☐ 4. Is the literature review comprehensive and accurate?
☐ 5. Are the objectives clear, unbiased, specific, consistent, and important?

## Methods: Patients and Research Setting

☐ 6. Are the patients selected and enrolled in the trial appropriately?
☐ 7. Are the inclusion and exclusion criteria used to select the trial patients appropriate, clear, and complete?
☐ 8. How closely does the trial sample represent the type of patient who will be treated with the investigational drug?
☐ 9. How similar are the trial drug therapy and regimen to that used in clinical practice?

## Methods: Use of Experimental Controls

☐10. Is the type of trial design used suitable?
☐11. Are the appropriate control groups used?
☐12. Is the patient assignment to the experimental and control groups randomized?
☐13. Are adequate blinding techniques used?

## Methods: Measurement of Results

☐14. Are the drug outcome measures clearly described and suitable?
☐15. Is the system of measuring the drug outcomes appropriate and adequately described?

## Results: Protocol and Data Management Problems

☐16. Are all protocol deviations reported and managed appropriately?
☐17. Are all missing data and patient withdrawals analyzed properly?

## Results: Presentation of Data

☐18. Are descriptive statistics used properly to describe the trial results?
☐19. How accurate and complete are the tables, figures, and graphs?

## Results: Interpretation of Data

☐20. Are the statistical comparisons between the investigational drug and the control treatment appropriate?
☐21. Are the differences reported between the investigational drug and the control treatment statistically significant and interpreted correctly?

## Discussion and Conclusions

☐22. Is a strong causal relationship established between the clinical outcome measured and the administration of the investigational drug?
☐23. Are the study results clinically important and generalizable to patients treated in the typical clinical practice setting?

# References

1. Brown ML. Cancer patient care in clinical trials sponsored by the National Cancer Institute: what does it cost? *J Nat Cancer Inst.* 1999; 91:847–53.

2. Brown GB. The changing audience for clinical trials. *Drug Info J.* 1995; 29:591–8.

3. Pathek DS, Escovitz A. Assuring the safe use of medications: the drug approval process and improving treatment decisions. *Clin Ther.* 1998; 20:C1–C4.

4. Alexander D. The pediatric pharmacology research unit network of the National Institute of Child Health and Human Development. *Drug Info J.* 1999; 33:385–91.

5. Pearson KC. Role of evidence-based medicine and clinical practice guidelines in treatment decisions. *Clin Ther.* 1998; 20:C80–C85.

6. Behrman RE. FDA approval of antiretroviral agents: an evolving paradigm. *Drug Info J.* 1999; 33:337–41.

7. Meyer RE, Griner PF, Wiessman J. Clinical research in medical schools: seizing the opportunity. *Proc Assoc Am Physicians.* 1998; 110:513–20.

8. Haynes RB, McKibbon KA, Fitzgerald D, et al. How to keep up with the medical literature II: deciding which journals to read regularly. *Ann Intern Med.* 1986; 105:309–12.

9. Woolf PK. Pressure to publish and fraud in science. *Ann Intern Med.* 1986; 104:254–6.

10. Thorn MD, Pulliam CC, Symons MJ, et al. Statistical and research quality of the medical and pharmacy literature. *Am J Hosp Pharm.* 1985; 42:1077–82.

11. Mosteller F, Gilbert JP, McPeek B. Reporting standards and research strategies. *Controlled Clin Trials.* 1980; 1:37–58.

12. Nahata MC. Publishing by pharmacists. *Drug Intell Clin Pharm.* 1989; 23:809–10.

13. Der Simonian R, Charette LJ, McPeek B, et al. Reporting on methods in clinical trials. *N Engl J Med.* 1982; 306:1332–7.

14. Newcombe RG. Towards a reduction in publication bias. *Br Med J.* 1987; 295:656–9.

15. Angell M. Publish or perish: a proposal. *Ann Intern Med.* 1986; 104:261–2.

16. Bailer JC. Science, statistics, and deception. *Ann Intern Med.* 1986; 104:259–60.

17. Huth EJ. Irresponsible authorship and wasteful publication. *Ann Intern Med.* 1986; 104:257–9.

18. Dickersin K, Min YI, Meinert CL. Factors influencing publication of research results. *JAMA.* 1992; 267:374–8.

19. Angell M, Relman AS. Fraud in biomedical research: a time for congressional restraint. *N Engl J Med.* 1988; 318:1462–3.

20. Conner CS. Conflicting data in the literature: a true dilemma. *Drug Intell Clin Pharm.* 1986; 20:444–5.

21. Horwitz RI. Complexity and contradiction in clinical trial research. *Am J Med.* 1987; 82:498–510.

22. Klimt CR. Varied acceptance of clinical trial results. *Controlled Clin Trials.* 1989; 10:135S–41S.

23. Haynes RB, Sackett DL, Tugwell P. Problems in the handling of clinical and research evidence by medical practitioners. *Arch Intern Med.* 1983; 143:1971–5.

24. Bennett KJ, Sackett DL, Haynes RB, et al. A controlled trial of teaching critical appraisal of the clinical literature to medical students. *JAMA.* 1987; 257:2451–4.

25. Brink CJ. Reading with a critical eye. *Am J Hosp Pharm.* 1986; 43:1697.

26. Clemens JD, Feinstein AR. Calcium carbonate and constipation: a historical review of medical mythopoeia. *Gastroenterol.* 1977; 72:957–61.

27. Rosenberg WM, Sackett DL. On the need for evidence-based medicine. *Therapie.* 1996; 51:212–7.

28. Sheiner L, Wakefield J. Population modeling in drug development. *Stat Methods Med Res.* 1999; 8:183–93.

29. Machado SG, Miller R, Hu C. A regulatory perspective on pharmacokinetic /pharmacodynamic modeling. *Stat Methods Med Res.* 1999; 8:217–45.

30. Lakings DB. Nonclinical drug development: pharmacology, drug

metabolism, and toxicology. In: Gaurino RA, ed. *New Drug Approval Process: The Global Challenge*. 3rd ed. New York: Marcel Dekker; 2000:17–54.31.

31. FDA Center for Drug Evaluation and Research. *From Test Tube to Patient: Improving Health Through Human Drugs*. Rockville MD: Food and Drug Administration; 1999:4–7.

32. Smith MC, Knapp DA. *Pharmacy, Drugs and Medical Care*. 5th ed. Baltimore: Williams and Wilkins; 1992:205–9.

33. Barnett-Parexel International Training Group. *An Overview of Drug Development*. San Diego: Barnett International; 1998:7–24.

34. FDA Center for Drug Evaluation and Research. *From Test Tube to Patient: Improving Health Through Human Drugs*. Rockville MD: Food and Drug Administration; 1999:33–40.

35. Shulman SR, Hewitt P, Manocchia M. Studies and inquiries into the FDA regulatory process: an historical review. *Drug Info J*. 1995; 29:385–414.

36. Kaitin KI, Brown JS. A drug lag update. *Drug Info J*. 1995; 29:361–75.

37. Lasagna L. Improving the drug development process. *Drug Info J*. 1995; 29:415–24.

38. DiMasi JA. Trends in drug development costs, times, and risks. *Drug Info J*. 1995; 29:375–84.

39. Cocchetto DM, Smiley L. The evolving paradigm for clinical development and regulatory approval of the antiretroviral drugs in the United States. *Drug Info J*. 1999; 33:357–62.

40. FDA Center for Drug Evaluation and Research. *From Test Tube to Patient: Improving Health Through Human Drugs*. Rockville MD: Food and Drug Administration; 1999:29–32.

41. FDA Center for Drug Evaluation and Research. *From Test Tube to Patient: Improving Health Through Human Drugs*. Rockville MD: Food and Drug Administration; 1999:14–7.

42. FDA Center for Drug Evaluation and Research. *From Test Tube to Patient: Improving Health Through Human Drugs*. Rockville MD: Food and Drug Administration; 1999:18–23.

43. Gaurino RA. Clinical research protocols. In: Gaurino RA, ed. *New Drug Approval Process: The Global Challenge*. 3rd ed. New York: Marcel Dekker; 2000:219–46.

44. Kirby D. Adverse drug events in clinical trials. In: Solgliero-Gilbert G, ed. *Drug Safety Assessment in Clinical Trials*. 3rd ed. New York: Marcel Dekker; 1993:25–38.

45. Gaurino RA. Adverse reactions and drug interactions of drugs. In: Gaurino RA, ed. *New Drug Approval Process: The Global Challenge*. 3rd ed. New York: Marcel Dekker; 2000:247–70.

46. Pally A, Berry SM. A decision analysis for an end of phase II go/stop decision. *Drug Info J*. 1999; 33:821–33.

47. Decoster G, Buyse M. Clinical research after drug approval: what is needed and what is not. *Drug Info J*. 1999; 33:627–34.

48. Hennessy S. Postmarketing drug surveillance: an epidemiologic approach. *Clin Ther*. 1998; 20:C32–9.

49. FDA Center for Drug Evaluation and Research. *From Test Tube to Patient: Improving Health Through Human Drugs*. Rockville MD: Food and Drug Administration; 1999:54–60.

50. Nahata MC. Pediatric drug formulations: a rate-limiting step. *Drug Info J*. 1999; 33:393–6.

51. Van Der Laan JW, Olejiniczak K. Pharmaceutical testing and pregnancy: from testing to labeling. *Drug Info J*. 1999; 33:1125–33.

52. Wilson JT. Questions and answers on labeling of drugs for children. *Drug Info J*. 1999; 33:375–83.

53. Golodner LF. The US Food and Drug Administration Modernization Act of 1997: impact on consumers. *Clin Ther*. 1998; 20:C20–5.

54. Janknegt RHYA. Postmarketing surveillance: applications and limitations, with special reference to the fluoroquinolones. In: Solgliero-Gilbert G, ed. *Drug Safety Assessment in Clinical Trials*. 3rd ed. New York: Marcel Dekker; 1993:415–26.

55. Pitts NE. Safety surveillance. In: Solgliero-Gilbert G, ed. *Drug Safety Assessment in Clinical Trials*. 3rd ed. New York: Marcel Dekker; 1993:331–414.

56. Bess AL. A successful global drug safety system: the Hoffmann–LaRoche experience. *Drug Info J*. 1999; 33:1109–16.

57. Laughren T. Premarketing studies in the drug approval process: understanding their limitations regarding the assessment of drug safety. *Clin Ther.* 1998; 20:C12–C19.

58. Ascione FJ, Manifold CC, Parenti MA. *Principles of Drug Information and Scientific Literature Evaluation.* Washington DC: American Pharmaceutical Association; 1994:57.

59. Moyne JT. Preclinical drug safety evaluation. In: Solgliero-Gilbert G, ed. *Drug Safety Assessment in Clinical Trials.* 3rd ed. New York: Marcel Dekker; 1993:1–24.

60. Elwood MJ. *Critical Appraisal of Epidemiological Studies and Clinical Trials.* New York: Oxford University Press; 1998:14–36.

61. Thapa PB, Gideon P, Cost T, et al. Antidepressants and the risk of falls among nursing home residents. *N Engl J Med.* 1998; 3339:875–82.

62. Strom BL. The promise of pharmacoepidemiology. *Ann Rev Pharmacol Toxicol.* 1987; 27:71–86.

63. Czeizel AE, Dudas I. Prevention of the first occurrence of neural-tube defects by periconceptional vitamin supplementation. *N Engl J Med.* 1992; 327:1832–5.

64. Bootman JL, Townsend RJ, McGhan WF. *Principles of Pharmacoeconomics.* Cincinnati: Harvey Whitney Books; 1991:3–17.

65. Sanchez LA. Applied pharmacoeconomics: evaluation and use of pharmacoeconomic data from literature. *Am J Health Sys Pharm.* 1999; 56:1630–40.

66. Bala AE, Kretschmer RAC, Gnann W, et al. Interpreting cost analyses of clinical interventions. *JAMA.* 1998; 279(1):54–7.

67. Guyatt GH, Heyting A, Jaeschke R, et al. N of 1 randomized trials for investigating new drugs. *Controlled Clin Trials.* 1990; 11:88–100.

68. Rochon J. A statistical model for the "n of 1" study. *J Clin Epidemiol.* 1990; 43:499–508.

69. Goldman S. Limitations and strengths of spontaneous reports data. *Clin Ther.* 1998; 20:C40–C58.

70. Yusuf S. Meta-analysis of randomized trials: looking back and looking ahead. *Controlled Clin Trials.* 1997; 18:594–601.

71. Koch GG, Schmid JE, Begun JM, et al. Meta-analysis of drug safety. In: Solgliero-Gilbert G, ed. *Drug Safety Assessment in Clinical Trials.* 3rd ed. New York: Marcel Dekker; 1993; 279–304.

72. Chen Y-T, Makuch RW. Use of meta-analysis to evaluate medical questions of interest: an application to studies of secondary prevention of acute myocardial infarction. *Drug Info J.* 1999; 33:1161–71.

73. Schmid CH. Exploring heterogeneity in randomized trials via meta-analysis. *Drug Info J.* 1999; 33:211–24.

74. Cappelleri JC, Ioannidis JPA, Schmid CH, et al. Large trials vs. meta-analysis of smaller trials: How do their results compare? *JAMA.* 1996; 276(16):1332–8.

75. Flather MD, Farkouh ME, Pogue JM, et al. Strength and limitations of meta-analysis. *Controlled Clin Trials.* 1997; 18:568–79.

76. Pocock SJ. *Clinical Trials: A Practical Approach.* New York: Wiley 1983:1–7.

77. Friedman LM, Furberg CD, DeMets DL. *Fundamentals of Clinical Trials.* 2nd ed. Littleton MA: PSG Publishing, 1985:ix.

78. Buck C, Donner A. The design of controlled experiments in the evaluation of non-therapeutic interventions. *J Chron Dis.* 1982; 35:531–8.

79. Barnes RW. Understanding investigative clinical trials. *J Vasc Surg.* 1989; 9:609–18.

80. Gehlbach SH. *Interpreting the Medical Literature: A Clinician's Guide.* New York: Macmillan, 1988:1–59.

81. Riegelman RK, Hirsch RP. *Studying a Study and Testing a Test.* 2nd ed. Boston: Little Brown, 1989:9–11.

82. Malone PM, Mosdell KW, Kier KL. *Drug Information: A Guide for Pharmacists.* Stamford: Appleton & Lange; 1996.

83. Smith GH, Norton LL, Ferrill MJ. *Evaluating Drug Literature: Module 2.* Bethesda MD: American Society of Health-System Pharmacists; 1995.

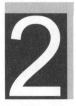

# Abstract and Introduction

➤❑ 1.  How clear and complete are the trial title and abstract?

➤❑ 2.  Is the article in a journal using a comprehensive review system to ensure quality?

➤❑ 3.  Are there important sources of biases in the author(s)' background or funding source?

➤❑ 4.  Is the literature review comprehensive and accurate?

➤❑ 5.  Are the study objectives clear, unbiased, specific, consistent, and important?

The primary purpose in reading an article describing a clinical drug trial is to learn more about how to use the drug effectively. To follow evidence-based practices, the healthcare practitioner needs to understand the scientific basis for the drug trial and the overall rationale for publishing the article. Thoroughly reading an article is difficult and time consuming. However, much can be learned from reading the study title, abstract, and introduction. This information is usually at the beginning of an article and can reveal a great deal about the purpose and focus of the trial, including the underlying motivation for its publication. In addition, understanding the mission of the journal in which the article is published, its system of reviewing manuscripts, and its sponsorship are also important.[1]

Unfortunately, many healthcare practitioners depend solely on the title and abstract and fail to read further. While good sources of summary information, the title and abstract are too limited and cannot provide sufficient insight into the research quality; therefore, they should not be used as the basis for clinical decision making.[1]

This chapter focuses on proper use of the study title, abstract, and introduction as sources of information about the clinical drug trial.

The journal and the publication process are covered. The five key questions (Questions 1–5) that should be addressed by the reader prior to reviewing the article are emphasized.

# ☑ 1. How clear and complete are the trial title and abstract?

The title and abstract are key because they are often the only source of information that the healthcare practitioner reviews. Thus, they should provide a clear, accurate, and comprehensive representation of content. Because of editorial and other space restrictions, this task is difficult, resulting in incomplete, misleading, or inaccurate information.

## Title

The title[1,2] is usually read first and is almost invariably located on the first page. Titles are usually the most common descriptive information listed in secondary and tertiary reference sources such as Medline and International Pharmaceutical Abstracts. Thus, clear, accurate, and unbiased titles are needed for proper assessment of the article's value.

Article titles are usually brief (often due to editorial restrictions) and should include[2]

- a concise description of the study,

- the listing of the primary authors and their affiliations (sometimes as a footnote), and

- appropriate keywords for indexing purposes in the major medical indices such as Medline.

The sponsor of the research, if any, is sometimes indicated as a footnote to the title. The title should be consistent with the information in the article abstract and should not include misleading or overstated claims (or conclusions).[2]

## Abstract

The abstract evolved from the old "summary and conclusions" section traditionally placed at the end of an article. It provides the reader with a timesaving and easy approach to reviewing a clinical drug trial. Its value as a quick source of information has become even more important with the availability of computerized information searching systems such as Medline and International Pharmaceutical Abstracts. In addition to the basic features of the article (e.g., authors, title, and journal), most computerized information systems provide brief summaries of the research. Those summaries are usually the article's abstract. Thus, it is important that the abstract clearly outlines the article's content.[1,3,4]

While the title is a brief guide to content, the abstract is intended to provide a concise summary of the clinical drug trial and is usually restricted to 200–400 words. A comprehensive abstract usually includes the purpose, research methodology, results, and the author's conclusions. While a complete description of the research conducted is important, the traditional abstract tends to focus on trial results.[3,4]

Comprehensive abstracts enable the reader to gain an understanding of the article's content and need to be written clearly. However, abstracts may be misleading because the research methodology and results sometimes cannot be sufficiently explained in the limited space allocated. In addition, abstracts are sometimes skewed by authors' tendency to describe the trial in the best possible manner. Thus, the value of a clinical drug trial should not be based on the abstract alone.[1,4–6]

The following example shows a traditional abstract format. This abstract was published in an article describing a clinical drug trial that compared astemizole, terfenadine, and placebo in the treatment of patients with hay fever.[7]

*In this double-blind study, 47 patients with hay fever were treated for eight days with either terfenadine 60 mg twice a day, astemizole 10 mg once a day, or placebo. On the second day of treatment terfenadine was statistically significantly superior to astemizole and placebo according to the ratings of symptomatology, efficacy and individual symptoms. The median onset of symptom alleviation was three hours for terfenadine and two days for astemizole. On the eighth day both astemizole and terfenadine were statistically more efficacious than placebo, but no significant differences were found between the two drugs. Both drugs were well tolerated.*

As shown, a major part of the abstract (about 70%) was devoted to the results. The remainder was a brief description of methodology, which included the number of subjects (47), the type of controls (double blind), duration of the study (eight days), and the dosages of the drugs to be compared. While the results were discussed in depth, the authors used vague terms such as "astemizole and terfenadine were more efficacious than placebo" and "both drugs were well tolerated" in describing their results. Neither the purpose of the study (i.e., to compare the therapeutic profiles of astemizole and terfenadine, including onset of action) nor the type of measures used were discussed in the abstract.

The need among healthcare practitioners for more summarized information generated a movement to urge journals to publish more structured and complete abstracts. In 1987, the Ad Hoc Working Group for the Critical Appraisal of the Medical Literature suggested dividing the abstract into the headings as shown in Table 2-1.[3,8–10]

**Table 2-1** Key Abstract Information[3]

| Heading | Description |
| --- | --- |
| **Objective** | The exact question addressed by the article |
| **Design** | The basic clinical drug trial design, including duration of follow-up |
| **Setting** | The location and type of care provided |
| **Patients/ participants** | Number of patients who entered and completed the trial, including how they were selected |
| **Interventions** | The essential features of the intervention, including the method of administration and duration of therapy |
| **Measurements/ results** | Important methods of assessing patients and key results reported |
| **Conclusions** | Important clinically relevant conclusions |

Some prominent health-related journals modified and adopted the structured abstract format. The following examples illustrate how the modified format is used to describe clinical drug trials published in the *Journal of the American Medical Association*[11] and the *New England Journal of Medicine.*[12]

The abstract from the *Journal of the American Medical Association*[11] describes a clinical drug trial that compared the toxicity (adverse upper GI effects) of two antiarthritic drugs (the nonsteroidal anti-inflammatory drugs and the cox-2 inhibitor rofecoxib) in patients with osteoarthritis.

**Context** *Nonsteroidal anti-inflammatory drug (NSAID-induced) gastrointestinal (GI) toxic effects, such as upper GI tract perforations, symptomatic gastroduodenal ulcers, and upper GI tract bleeding (PUBs), are thought to be attributable to cyclooxygenase 1 (COX-1) inhibition. Rofecoxib specifically inhibits COX-2 and has demonstrated a low potential for causing upper GI injury.*

**Objective** *To compare the incidence of PUBs in patients with osteoarthritis treated with rofecoxib vs NSAIDS.*

**Design** *Pre-specified analysis of all 8 double-blind, randomized phase 2b/3 rofecoxib osteoarthritis trials conducted from December 1996 through March 1998, including one 6-week dose-ranging study, two 6-week efficacy studies vs ibuprofen and placebo, two 1-year efficacy studies vs diclofenac, two 6-month endoscopy studies vs ibuprofen and placebo, and one 6-week efficacy study vs nabumetone and placebo.*

**Setting** *Multinational sites.*

**Participants** *Osteoarthritis patients (N = 5435; mean age, 63 years [range, 38-94 years]; 72.9% women).*

*Interventions Rofecoxib, 12.5, 25, or 50 mg/d (n = 1209, 1603, and 545, respectively, combined) vs ibuprofen, 800 mg 3 times per day (n = 847), diclofenac, 50 mg 3 times per day (n = 590); or nabumetone, 1500 mg/d (n = 127) (combined).*

**Main Outcome Measure** *Cumulative incidence of PUBs for rofecoxib vs NSAIDS, based on survival analysis of time to first PUB diagnosis, using PUBs that met pre-specified criteria judged by a blinded, external adjudication committee.*

**Results** *The incidence of PUBs over 12 months was significantly lower with rofecoxib vs NSAIDs (12-month cumulative incidence, 1.3% vs 1.8%; P = .046; rate per 100 patient-years, 1.33 vs 2.60; relative risk, 0.51; 95% confidence interval, 0.26-1.00). The cumulative incidence of dyspeptic GI adverse experiences was also lower with rofecoxib vs NSAIDS over 6 months (23.5% vs 25.5%; P = .02), after which the incidence rates converged.*

**Conclusion** *In a combined analysis of 8 trials of patients with osteoarthritis, treatment with rofecoxib was associated with a significantly lower incidence of PUBs than treatment with NSAIDS.*

As shown, the abstract is divided into nine headings, in which only one includes results. Compared to the traditional abstract, significantly more information is provided about the design and methods. In addition, the abstract is structured so that the reader can easily identify relevant information.

The *New England Journal of Medicine*[12] abstract is less structured and is divided into fewer headings. Unlike the *JAMA* abstract, only four headings are used, with the primary difference being that the various method components are summarized under one heading. A typical abstract is one that describes the use of metronidazole to prevent preterm delivery in pregnant women with asymptomatic bacterial vaginosis.[12]

**Background**. *Bacterial vaginosis has been associated with preterm birth. In clinical trials, the treatment of bacterial vaginosis in pregnant women who previously had a preterm delivery reduced the risk of recurrence.*

**Methods.** *To determine whether treating women in a general obstetrical population who have asymptomatic bacterial vaginosis (as diagnosed on the basis of vaginal Gram's staining and pH) prevents preterm delivery, we randomly assigned 1953 women who were 16 to less than 24 weeks pregnant to receive two 2-g doses of metronidazole or placebo. The diagnostic studies were repeated and a second treatment was administered to all the women at 24 to less than 30 weeks' gestation. The primary outcome was the rate of delivery before 37 weeks' gestation.*

**Results**. *Bacterial vaginosis resolved in 657 of 845 women who had follow-up Gram's staining in the metronidazole group (77.8* *percent) and 321 of 859 women in the placebo group (37.4 percent). Data on the time and characteristics of delivery were available for 953 women in the metronidazole group and 966 in the placebo group. Preterm delivery occurred in 116 women in the metronidazole group (12.2 percent) and 121 women in the placebo group (12.5 percent) (relative risk, 1.0; 95 percent confidence interval, 0.8 to 1.2). Treatment did not prevent preterm deliveries that resulted from spontaneous labor (5.1 percent in the metronidazole group vs. 5.7 percent in the placebo group) or spontaneous rupture of the membranes (4.2 percent vs. 3.7 percent), nor did it prevent delivery before 32 weeks (2.3 percent vs. 2.7 percent). Treatment with metronidazole did not reduce the occurrence of preterm labor, intraamniotic or postpartum infections, neonatal sepsis, or admission of the infant to the neonatal intensive care unit.*

***Conclusions****. The treatment of asymptomatic bacterial vaginosis in pregnant women does not reduce the occurrence of preterm delivery or other adverse perinatal outcomes.*

The use of more structured abstracts appears to overcome some limitations of the traditional abstract as a source of information. However, even well-designed overviews often do not synthesize information about the benefits, risks, and costs of drug therapy in a way that facilitates clinical decision making.[13,14]

# ☑ 2. Is the article in a journal using a comprehensive review system to ensure quality?

Although many abstracts provide sufficient information, most practitioners lack either the time or expertise to make such judgments on quality. Quite often, the practitioner relies on the type of journal in which the article is published to determine research quality. Thus, the process in which the journal selects articles to publish is an important mechanism to ensure quality.

Most journal editors use a systematic process and a predetermined set of criteria to determine which articles submitted for publication are published. Although some articles are authored by the editorial staff of the journal or solicited from writers not on staff, most journal articles are selected from those voluntarily submitted by independent authors. Thus, a journal's reputation is partially based on the process and the criteria that it uses to select articles for publication.

## Peer Review

The most important part of the journal selection process is the use of a peer review system. Peer review is defined as "the assessment by experts (peers) of the material submitted for publication in scientific and technical periodicals." Although the system is imperfect, most editors believe that it provides the best mechanism by which submitted manuscripts can be improved, regardless of whether they are published in the journal to which they were originally submitted.[15,16]

The peer review system for examining scientific communications has existed for a long time, although the formalized system in existence today is relatively new. Frequently, credit for introducing the philosophy of peer review is assigned to the Royal Society of London, which introduced the concept of scientific review of manuscripts in 1752. However, other scholars suggested that the system started almost 100 years earlier with the introduction of the first "scientific journal" in 1665. Despite the controversy about its origin, the peer review system has evolved in an unsystematic fashion to the current, almost universally accepted system. The universal implementation was needed to handle the large numbers of articles submitted for publication after World War II and to meet the demands of an increasingly specialized scientific community.[17,18]

Although varying by journal, the typical peer review system consists of the journal editor(s) sending manuscripts to one or more "experts" for review and comment on the research methodology and the clinical significance of the findings. The peer reviewers, who are usually anonymous to the article authors, typically make independent recommendations to accept, revise, or reject a manuscript for publication. The journal editor usually examines the reviews and decides the final action for the manuscript, often in consultation with associate editors or the editorial staff.[19,20]

The peer review system has two general goals:

- to ensure that methodologically sound research articles are published and

- to introduce into clinical practice research findings that will improve the quality of patient care.

The process is most effective when it accomplishes the following specific objectives:[15, 21,22]

- Screens out poorly conceived, designed, or executed reports of investigations.

- Ensures proper consideration and recognition of other relevant work.

- Leads to helpful revisions and consequent improvements in the quality of manuscripts reviewed.

- Aids in steering research results to the most appropriate journals.

- Raises the technical quality of the field by improving the training, education, and motivation of research scientists.

- Puts a stamp of quality on individual papers as an aid to non-experts who may use the results.

- Improves professional acceptance and approval of journals.

Although it is the best method to ensure that scientifically valid and important research findings are published, the peer review system is limited by the lack of clear standards and criteria for peer reviewers to use when evaluating journal articles. While there appears to be a consensus regarding the recommendation to accept a manuscript, reviewers often disagree on what parts of a manuscript need revision. Disagreements commonly occur over

- the quality of the writing,

- the overall presentation of the research,

- the appropriateness of the statistical analysis, or

- the type of references used.

Some reviewers submit reviews of poor quality, placing more pressure on the editors to decide whether or not to accept the manuscript.[22-27]

Peer review systems are usually not successful in preventing multiple publication of the same article or narrowed subsets of the same research. Scientific fraud is equally difficult to detect. It is also possible that the peer review process may restrict the introduction of innovative ideas that could eventually lead to improvements in patient care, commonly called "publication bias."[15,22,28-34]

Publication bias is often defined as the tendency to publish trials showing the advantages of new treatments and to not publish studies finding no such advantages. Although strong evidence to support this claim is lacking, the consequences would be important because practitioners could only find literature biased toward positive results. Journals might offset these biases with changes such as a careful monitoring of the review process, encouraging the publishing of sound methodological studies with "negative" results, and establishing policies that allow a fair appeal process for a rejected manuscript.[33-35]

## Journal Editorial Boards

Journals often have editorial boards[36] consisting of individuals who screen manuscripts prior to peer review or perform the peer review themselves. They also function as advisors to the editor on overall journal policy. Reputable journals have editorial boards composed of well-known researchers and leaders in their respective disciplines. Their backgrounds may differ depending on the journal. Boards of journals with a broad clinical focus should have members from a wide range of disciplines, and those of specialty journals should include well-respected members of the discipline. The editorial board usually is listed on or near the title page of each issue. Some journals, however, recruit well-known individuals to serve on the board for prestigious reasons without seeking their advice.[36]

# ☑ 3. Are there important sources of biases in the author(s)' background or funding source?

One key component to assessing the quality of the results involves determining the extent to which the author(s) design and interpret the study in a biased manner. The reason for this concern is the subtle effect that investigator bias can have on the trial design or interpretation of its results. Investigator bias is often defined as a prejudice or partiality for a certain outcome (usually positive results) that may or may not be conscious. Where no prejudice exists, investigator bias is arbitrary compared to systematic bias. Investigator bias is unpredictable, whereas systematic bias can be detected and managed through design changes or statistical analysis.[31]

Investigator bias can be large or subtle, but in either case it can have a substantial impact on the trial. Some investigators may have great confidence that the drug therapy will work and are enthusiastic to prove it. Unless their bias is offset by the design of the trial, investigators can affect the study results by how they

- enroll the study subjects,

- evaluate the success of the investigational drug, and

- interpret the study results.

Because such bias can damage a trial, every effort should be made to eliminate it in the design, conduct, and analysis. Investigator bias is difficult to detect, even after careful examination of the study design. However, a useful approach is to examine the author(s)' background, the study site, and the source of funding for the study.[31]

## Author(s)' Background

The purpose of examining the author(s)' credentials is to assess the research team's competence to conduct a properly designed clinical drug trial and to interpret the results correctly. In a clinical trial, the competence of investigators and staff usually needs to be justified prior to trial initiation by the funding agency, either federal or private. Also, investigator qualifications may be demonstrated by past performance in similar trials. One important competency is the investigator's ability to recruit eligible participants. Another factor is the ability to deliver the drug therapy as specified in the protocol while providing the best care for participants and to keep participants in the study. Establishing an appropriate data collection and management system is also important.[31,37]

The most common source of information to assess the author(s)' competence is in the study title. Usually, the author is listed immediately below the title and in most publications of clinical drug trials more than one author is listed. The primary author, however, is listed first and usually is the person in charge of conducting the study as well as writing the article. This individual is typically the principal investigator. The remaining authors are either listed in alphabetical order, as if all had equal responsibility for the study and article, or in order of responsibility. The primary purpose of listing the authors is to inform the healthcare practitioner of the research team's credentials. Some journals list the authors' degrees after their names, and other journals include degrees at the bottom of the title page.[38–40]

The credentials of the authors should be reviewed carefully to evaluate their ability to properly conduct and complete the clinical drug trial. Unfortunately, only a small amount of information is usually provided, primarily because of editorial restrictions. Usually, just the investigators' educational background (degrees held), employer, and employment position are provided. Despite the limited amount of information available, some judgments can be made. For example, a study conducted in the area of cancer chemotherapy should have one or more investigators with advanced training in that specialty. It is often helpful to have a biostatistician involved in the study because it may lend more credibility to the study's design and analysis. While information about authors is important, it is often incomplete. A few journals do not list complete credentials of authors, and many journals do not indicate if they are specialists.[41]

Another source of assessing the authors' competence is their past research. Authors with a publication record that involves similar research should have the experience needed to complete the relatively complex study designs of most clinical drug trials. The relevant publication experience of the author can sometimes be found in the literature review section of the article or, more often, through a computerized search of medical literature databases such as Medline. However, competent performance in one trial does not guarantee the same in the next.[38]

The authors' past experience, training, and previous performance are useful but indirect measures of their competence at performing the clinical drug trial. Perhaps the best proof may be completing the current drug trial and getting it published in a respected peer review journal.[31]

## Study Location

A potential source of bias is the location of the clinical drug trial, often related to the source of funding. Some funding for clinical drug research comes from organizations such as the federal government (e.g., the National Institutes of Health), private foundations (e.g., the American Heart

Association), or professional organizations (e.g., the American Society of Health-System Pharmacists). The location of this type of research is typically the academic health center or a large healthcare organization.[42,43]

The primary source of funding for clinical drug research is the pharmaceutical manufacturer. A great deal of that research is done on a contractual basis with commercial organizations called contract review organizations (CROs). According to one estimate, the percentage of studies sponsored by the manufacturer that includes a contract research component has increased from 28% in 1993 to 64% in 1998. It was estimated that, in 1999, approximately 450 CROs existed in the United States and Europe.[44,45]

The clinical aspects of the drug approval process are labor intensive and costly. Thus, it is not surprising that the manufacturer contracts to outside sources. Typically, because the entire clinical testing program spans several years and many different types of studies, the manufacturer uses multiple CROs for different services. The CRO is more involved in the implemention of the Clinical Development Plan than in the overall development program. The type of work contracted depends on the sponsor. In some instances, it involves all aspects of a particular study. In other situations, only specific services such as data analysis or pharmacokinetic evaluation are contracted to support the research done by the sponsor's staff. Most contracts deal with one or more of the most labor-intensive portions of clinical research, namely the clinical monitoring of study sites, data entry, programming for data listings and summary tables, and writing clinical study reports.[45]

While manufacturer use of CROs has been successful, problems are associated with the relationship. Time delays in producing the desired result, miscommunication between the sponsor and the CRO, and sloppy data management occur. The traditional collaborative process between the sponsor and the CRO has not resulted in substantial improvement in the clinical development time, despite improvement in the regulatory review process. This continual time lag resulted in the development of Site Management Organizations (SMOs), which are business enterprises with multiple study locations (regional, national, and international) that offer a full range of services to the manufacturer. They focus on providing two primary assets: a large and diverse group of physicians and patients and a thorough, comprehensive data collection system. In 1999, it was estimated that there were 30–40 SMOs in the European and United States marketplace, most privately owned. The long-term success of the SMOs in clinical drug development is not known, but it is anticipated that they will be useful because of their ability to provide a wider range of information more efficiently.[44,46,47]

Academic medical centers are traditional sources of manufacturer-contracted clinical research because of their patient base and clinical experts. Although slow to adapt to the current operating demands of drug sponsors, these institutions are modifying their practices to act more like CROs and SMOs.[46,48]

Although all organizations with a commercial interest in drug development must comply with strict regulatory requirements in completing clinical drug trials, the potential for bias exists. Thus, when examining trial results, healthcare practitioners need to be aware of where the study was produced. Unfortunately, this information is often not given or is incomplete or unclear. If presented, the information is usually found in the title or as a footnote. The relevant locations involved (institutions, universities, and other medical offices) should be described, and the names, addresses, and telephone numbers for all test laboratories involved in the study should be given.[41]

## Potential Conflict of Interest

Dealing with a researcher's potential financial conflict of interest[31,49–52] in publishing study findings is one of the most contentious issues in biomedical research. There is a wide range of potential conflicts among researchers, but the most important is in the area of financial support or gifts from the pharmaceutical manufacturer. A conflict of interest is a set of circumstances whereby the researcher's interpretation of the trial findings is unduly influenced by the financial support received from the drug manufacturer. The financial support itself is not considered inappropriate. Rather, the concern is about the extent that the support dominates the investigator's interpretation.

Many journals, beginning with the *New England Journal of Medicine* in 1984, deal with the increasing influence of commercialism in biomedical support by instituting policies in which the authors disclose any business associations that could affect their research. The advantage of full disclosure is that it gives the reader information needed to decide about the interpretation of the study results. Unfortunately, full disclosure only indicates that a potential conflict of interest exists; it does not do much to resolve any potential bias. Thus, more stringent measures have been suggested, such as abstention (withdrawal from authorship), divestiture (removal of the financial support, if possible), or prohibition (nonparticipation in research areas in which a financial arrangement exists).[52]

Financial arrangements or potential conflicts of interests of the authors are usually found in the first part of the article, often as a footnote. Sources of funding for the research are commonly provided, and sometimes other financial arrangements are disclosed.

# ☑ 4. Is the literature review comprehensive and accurate?

The literature review or background section usually is at the beginning of the article, often just after the abstract and title, and describes the rationale for drug trial. The utility of the literature review can be assessed by examining its content, the references used, and the quality of the citation process.[53]

## Content

The literature review[2,41] should cover past research, including a brief discussion of the history of treating the disorder, the relative efficacy of previous drug therapy, and any clinical drug trials that compared the new drug with the existing standard drug treatment. The abstract is a good source of information about the clinical drug trial, but the literature review is the best place to begin assessment of the quality of the reported research. It should demonstrate that the benefits found in the current study will likely outweigh the risks to patients. This objective is important because healthcare practitioners should be encouraged to read only those studies that have the potential to improve patient care.

The ideal literature review should be a summary of previous knowledge about the investigational drug and general treatment for the disease. A critical discussion of the strengths and weaknesses of previous studies might be included to assure the reader that these mistakes will be avoided in the current clinical drug trial and that further study is justified. The natural history of the disease and its treatment should be described succinctly. The identity and potency of the drug(s) being used may be given as well as the study setting (e.g., nursing homes, psychiatric wards, outpatient clinics) and the rationale for using that setting. Authors should avoid citing only their own past research when providing background information because of a potential for a biased perspective. All major statements in the literature review should be supported by references.[2,41]

The literature review is important information for healthcare practitioners who lack time to read the primary literature. Unfortunately, journal space considerations limit its relative size. Thus, most literature reviews do not provide a complete discussion of the past research, although an extensive list of references may be supplied.

## References

The references used by the author to establish the basis of the literature review are generally cited in the text but placed in the last section of the article. Although citation styles vary, most biomedical journals follow the standards outlined in the document entitled "Uniform Requirements for Manuscripts Submitted to Biomedical Journals." While the reference style is relatively standardized, authors vary in their use of references and the quality of their citations.[54]

Evaluating the references used to support the literature review indirectly assesses the quality of the literature review and the author's understanding of previous research. There are several key areas to examine. One area is the number of references cited. The number usually indicates how thoroughly the literature was reviewed. Most references should be to original articles describing previous clinical drug trials, including recently published articles. However, in some cases, one or two classic references may be appropriate. References to abstracts, unpublished observations, and personal communications should be avoided or at least be a small part of the reference list. Articles with reference lists that include only citations of books or reviews may indicate a lack of critical evaluation of past research. If the authors cite only their work, the article reference list may be too narrow and biased.[2]

Of course, to confirm that the authors completely reviewed the literature, healthcare practitioners could perform their own search. This process, however, is time consuming and not likely to occur. Thus, healthcare practitioners are often forced to decide about the quality of the review and its thoroughness based on relatively limited information.

Although the lack of a complete discussion of past research can mislead the healthcare practitioner, the amount of supportive research can also be misrepresented by citing redundant or repetitive publications. Redundant publications contain essentially the same material published in another journal article. Publication of redundant articles is discouraged by most journals, but this effort is difficult to enforce.

Repetitive articles are similar to redundant articles in that they involve publishing essentially the same material in more than one type of publication. The major difference is that repetitive articles involve material published more often and in a variety of sources such as original research articles, book chapters, abstracts, or review articles.

Divided articles involve splitting the findings of a single research project into a string of publications. While this practice may be appropriate in some cases, the effort sometimes is solely to lengthen the investigator's publication record.[28,55]

Articles are occasionally retracted because of unintentional research errors (rarely) or fraudulent data or ideas. Unfortunately, retracted articles often continue to be cited by other investigators. One investigation[56] identified 82 retracted studies published from 1970 to 1989. These studies were cited an average of nine times after the article was retracted.

Another problem area in the literature review involves incorrect or imprecise use of the references. These problems can be divided into citation errors and quotation errors.

Citation errors occur when certain facts about the referenced article are incorrectly listed. These facts include the author's name, article title, or the journal source. Major citation errors are often defined as those that prevent easy and immediate identification of the source of the reference and include

- incorrect journal name,

- omission of the volume or year of the publication, or

- incorrect page numbers.

In contrast, minor citation errors do not prevent location of the citation and consist of incorrect author initials or page numbers of the article.

Citation error rates appear to be high, ranging from 24% to 48%. Major errors are reported to occur in approximately 3–9% of cited references.[43,57,58]

Quotation errors occur when the intent of the cited clinical drug trial is distorted. A major quotation error is one in which the cited reference fails to substantiate, or even contradicts, the statements made in the literature review section. Minor quotation errors do not significantly distort the research findings but tend to oversimplify the conclusions. Quotation errors occur slightly less often than citation errors, with reported incidence rates of 15–30%. Major quotation errors reportedly occur in 6–27% of cited references.[43,57,58]

Citation or quotation errors frustrate the healthcare practitioner trying to locate the source or may create a negative impression about the investigators' attention to details. Use of misleading or improper references (e.g., redundant, repetitive, divided, or retracted publications) is more difficult to detect and can lead the unfamiliar healthcare practitioner to give more credibility to a statement than it may deserve. Referencing errors may cause the user to doubt the quality of the investigators' preparation, suggesting that references to prior work were not consulted or personally reviewed but merely cited or copied from another article.[53]

# ☑ 5. Are the study objectives clear, unbiased, specific, consistent, and important?

The study objectives are usually placed just after the background section and should represent the author(s)' beliefs regarding the expected effect of the experimental drug. The objectives usually consist of one to five concise statements that summarize the research methodology, including the expected outcome of the trial. Appropriate objectives are important because they provide a guide to the suitability of the clinical drug trial and how to measure its success (*see* Chapter 8, Question 20). Thus, study objectives are necessary for a thorough evaluation. The objectives should be clearly stated or the purpose of the investigation may not be clear. Poorly stated or inadequate objectives make it difficult to read and evaluate clinical studies and may be a reflection of poor study design or poor conduction of the trial. The objectives should clearly describe the trial hypotheses, which are defined as the expected relationships to be measured in the trial or the primary questions to be addressed.[5,41,59]

## Quality

Evaluation of the objectives involves assessing their clarity, objectivity, specificity, value, and consistency with the investigators' conclusions. They should explicitly state

■ the purpose of the clinical research project,

- the type of study (i.e., open, double blind, crossover),
- a brief description of the medications used,
- the outcome measures, and
- the type of patient population to be evaluated.

Clear objectives often indicate a strong research plan and are easy to evaluate.[41,60]

This example of a clear objective is from a clinical drug trial[61] that assessed the efficacy of felbamate for seizure control:

> *The objective of this study was to evaluate the efficacy and safety of felbamate under double-blind conditions in patients with refractory partial-onset seizures with or without generalizations who had completed a hospital evaluation for epilepsy surgery.*

This objective clearly states what is planned. The description includes the type of patient studied, research setting and design, and drug effects measured.

The study objectives and the outcome measures must be relevant and logical. The clinical drug trial should be ignored if the objective appears to focus on providing marginally useful information for the standard drug treatment of the illness.[1,59]

## Multiple Objectives

Many clinical drug trials are so costly that investigators often try to test more than one objective to obtain as much information as possible. The use of multiple objectives[62–68] is appropriate if limited in number and clearly distinguished from each other.

The major problem with multiple objectives is the increased probability of identifying false differences between the investigational drug and the control treatment. This problem is particularly evident when the differences are not significant only on measures of the secondary objectives. In fact, some biostatisticians suggest that the observed differences on measures of the secondary objectives only cannot be properly interpreted and analyzed and thus should be ignored.[65]

One approach is to use more rigid statistical criteria for testing the secondary objective. Other strategies include defining a single primary outcome, adjusting for multiple testing, combining data from multiple endpoints into a single global statistic, adopting a combined endpoint, or exploring all outcomes with equal interest.[62,64–67]

One study[67] with multiple objectives compared the effects of dolasetron and ondansetron on acute and delayed nausea and vomiting after chemotherapy:

*The objectives of the trial were as follows: (1) to compare the efficacy of ondansetron and dolasetron in controlling nausea and vomiting in the first 24 hours; (2) to evaluate whether dexamethasone adds to the antiemetic efficacy of dolasetron and ondansetron in the first 24 hours and (3) to extend these comparisons (i.e., dolasetron and ondansetron with or without dexamethasone) over 7 days. A fourth objective was to determine whether 5 $HT_1$ antagonists add to the antiemetic efficacy of dexamethasone in the delayed phase (days 2 to 7); results from this component of the trial have been reported separately.*

The first objective is the primary one, while objectives 2–4 are related but secondary. While related, there may be too many objectives for one study.

A clinical drug trial that includes multiple but vaguely connected objectives suggests poor research methodology. The investigators may allocate too much attention to achieving their multiple objectives rather than focusing on the primary question. Here's an example of a vaguely connected set of objectives in a clinical drug trial of the effectiveness of trimethoprim–sulfamethoxazole for acute bronchitis.[69]

The primary objective was:

*Patients treated with trimethoprim and sulfamethoxazole would have a shorter duration of illness as measured by cough, sputum production, fever, and general sense of well-being.*

and the secondary objective read:

*that performing sputum gram stains would allow a more accurate prediction of subjects who would benefit from antibiotic drug therapy.*

The secondary objective suggests that the investigators may have gotten too broad in their research plan because it is not closely related to the primary objective. It is also possible that the trial objectives changed during the project, introducing more bias into the reporting of results.

# References

1. Sackett DL. How to read clinical journals: I. Why to read them and how to start reading them critically. *CMA J.* 1981; 124:555–8.

2. Berzon RA. Understanding and using health-related quality of life instruments within clinical research studies. In: Staquet MJ, Hays RD, Fayers PM, eds. *Quality of Life Assessment in Clinical Trials.* New York: Oxford University Press; 1998:3–15.

3. Ad Hoc Working Group for Critical Appraisal of the Medical Literature. A proposal for more informative abstracts of clinical articles. *Ann Intern Med.* 1987; 106:598–604.

4. Cuddy PG, Elenbaas RM, Elenbaas JK. Evaluating the medical literature. Part I: abstract, introduction, methods. *Ann Emerg Med.* 1983; 12:549–55.

5. Friedman LM, Furberg CD, DeMets DL. *Fundamentals of Clinical Trials.* Littleton, MA: PSG Publishing, 1985: 11, 236.

6. Gehlbach SH. *Interpreting the Medical Literature: A Clinician's Guide.* Lexington, MA: DC Heath, 1982:6–8.

7. Girard JP, Sommacal-Schopf D, Bibliardi P, et al. Double-blind comparison of astemizole, terfenadine and placebo in hay fever with special regard to onset of action. *J Int Med Res.* 1985; 13:102–8.

8. Rennie D, Glass RM. Structuring abstracts to make them more informative. *JAMA.* 1991; 266:116–7.

9. Francioli P, Etienne J, Hoigne R, et al. Treatment of streptococcal endocarditis with a single daily dose of ceftriaxone sodium for 4 weeks. *JAMA.* 1992; 267:264–7.

10. Classen DC, Evans RS, Pestotnik SL, et al. The timing of prophylactic administration of antibiotics and the risk of surgical-wound infection. *N Engl J Med.* 1992; 326:281–6.

11. Langman MJ, Jensen DM, Watson DJ, et al. Adverse upper gastrointestinal effects of rofecoxib compared with NSAIDS. *JAMA.* 1999; 282:1929–33.

12. Carey JC, Klebanoff MA, Hauth JC, et al. Metronidazole to prevent preterm delivery in pregnant women with asymptomatic bacterial vaginosis. *N Engl J Med.* 2000; 342(8):534–40.

13. Haynes RB, Mulrow CD, Huth EJ, et al. More informative abstracts revisted. *Cleft Palate-Craniofacial J.* 1996; 33(1):1–9.

14. Hayward RSA, Wilson MC, Tunis SR, et al. More informative abstracts of articles describing clinical practice guidelines. *Am Coll Physicians.* 1993; 118:731–7.

15. Bailar JC, Patterson K. Journal peer review: the need for a research agenda. *N Engl J Med.* 1985; 312:654–7.

16. Wienberger M, Tierney WM, Avanian JZ, et al. The role of peer-reviewed journals in science. *Med Care.* 2000; 38:1–3.

17. Burnham JC. The evolution of editorial peer review. *JAMA.* 1990; 263:1323–9.

18. Kronick DA. Peer review in 18th-century scientific journalism. *JAMA.* 1990; 263:1321–2.

19. Morgan PP. Author, editor and reviewer: how manuscripts become journal articles. *CMA J.* 1981; 124:664–6.

20. Weller AC. Editorial peer review in U.S. medical journals. *JAMA.* 1990; 263:1344–7.

21. Cantekin EI, McGuire TW, Potter RL. Biomedical information, peer review, and conflict of interest as they influence public health. *JAMA.* 1990; 263:1427–30.

22. Horrobin DF. The philosophical basis of peer review and the suppression of innovation. *JAMA.* 1990; 263:1438–41.

23. Garfunkel JM, Ulshen MH, Hamrick HJ, et al. Problems identified by secondary review of accepted manuscripts. *JAMA.* 1990; 263:1369–71.

24. Stossel TP. Reviewer status and review quality: experience of the journal of clinical investigation. *N Engl J Med.* 1985; 312:658–60.

25. Crigger NJ. What we owe the author: rethinking editorial peer review. *Nursing Ethics.* 1998; 5(5):451–8.

26. Lock S, Smith J. What do peer reviewers do? *JAMA.* 1990; 263:1341–3.

27. Cleary JD, Alexander B. Blinded versus nonblind review: a reevaluation of selected medical journals. *Drug Intell Clin Pharm.* 1990; 24:1117–8.

28. Angell M, Relman AS. Redundant publication. *N Engl J Med.* 1989; 320:1212–4.

29. Angell M, Relman AS. How good is peer review? *N Engl J Med.* 1989; 321:827–9.

30. Stehbens WE. Basic philosophy and concepts underlying scientific peer review. *Med. Hypotheses.* 1999; 52(1):31–6.

31. DeMets D. Distinction between fraud, bias, errors, misunderstanding, and incompetence. *Controlled Clin Trials.* 1997; 18:637–50.

32. Ioannides JP, Cappelleri JC, Sacks HS, et al. The relationship between study design, results, and reporting of randomized clinical trials of HIV infection. *Controlled Clin Trials.* 1997; 18:431–44.

33. Chalmers TC, Frank CS, Reitman D. Minimizing the three stages of publication bias. *JAMA.* 1990; 263:1392–5.

34. Sharp DW. What can and should be done to reduce publication bias? The perspective of an editor. *JAMA.* 1990; 263:1390–1.

35. Dickersin K, Min Y, Meinert CL. Factors influencing publication of research results. *JAMA.* 1992; 267:374–8.

36. Boldt J, Maleck W. Composition of editorial/advisory boards of major English-language anesthesia/critical care journals. *Acta Anesth Scand.* 2000; 44:175–9.

37. Mackintosh DR. Detection of negligence, fraud, and other bad faith efforts during field auditing of clinical trial sites. *Drug Info J.* 1996; 30:645–53.

38. Emden C. Establishing a "track record": research productivity and nursing academe. *Aust J Adv Nursing.* 1998; 16:29–33.

39. Niemcryk SJ, Glascoff DW. Considerations in presenting, interpreting, and reviewing research findings. *J Transplant Coordination.* 1997; 7:41–5.

40. Gaeta TJ. Authorship: "Law" and order. *Acad Emerg Med.* 1999; 6:297–301.

41. Gaurino RA. Clinical research protocols. In: Gaurino RA, ed. *New Drug Approval Process: The Global Challenge.* 3rd ed. New York: Marcel Dekker; 2000:219–46.

42. Hillman AJ, Eisenberg JM, Pauly MV, et al. Avoiding bias in the conduct and reporting of cost-effectiveness research sponsored by pharmaceutical companies. *N Engl J Med.* 1991; 324:1362–5.

43. Pocock SJ. *Clinical Trials: A Practical Approach.* New York: Wiley, 1983:240.

44. Maloff BL. Partnering for success in performance measurements for sponsors, contract research organizations, and site management organizations. *Drug Info J.* 1999; 33:655–61.

45. Lakings DB, Mancinin ADJ. Working with a CRO. In: Gaurino RA, ed. *New Drug Approval Process: The Global Challenge.* 3rd ed. New York: Marcel Dekker; 2000:439–63.

46. Getz K. The evolving SMO in the United States. In: Gaurino RA, ed. *New Drug Approval Process: The Global Challenge.* 3rd ed. New York: Marcel Dekker; 2000:455–63.

47. Lewis NJ. Keys to successful outsourcing choices. *Contract Pharma.* 2000; January/February:38–43.

48. Meyer RE, Griner PF, Wiessman J. Clinical research in medical schools:seizing the opportunity. *Proc Assoc Am Physicians.* 1998; 110:513–20.

49. Thompson DF. Understanding financial conflicts of interest. *N Engl J Med.* 1993; 329:573–6.

50. Kassirer JP, Angell M. Financial conflict of interest in biomedical research. *N Engl J Med.* 1993; 329:570–1.

51. Price VH. Author's conflicts of interest: A disclosure and editors' reply. *N Engl J Med.* 1999; 341:1618–9.

52. Angell M, Utiger RD, Wood AJJ. Disclosure of author's conflicts of interest: A follow-up. *N Engl J Med.* 2000; 342(8):586–7.

53. Neihouse PF, Priske SC. Quotation accuracy in review articles. *Drug Intell Clin Pharm.* 1989; 23:594–6.

54. Anonymous. Uniform requirements for manuscripts submitted to biomedical journals. *N Engl J Med.* 1997; 336:309–15.

55. Huth EJ. Irresponsible authorship and wasteful publication. *Ann Intern Med.* 1986; 104:257–9.

56. Pfeifer MP, Snodgrass GL. The continued use of retracted, invalid scientific literature. *JAMA.* 1990; 263:1420–3.

57. Eichorn P, Yankauer A. Do authors check their references? A survey of accuracy of references in three public health journals. *Am J Public Health.* 1987; 77:1011–2.

58. Evans JT, Nadjari HI, Burchell SA. Quotational and reference accuracy in surgical journals. *JAMA.* 1990; 263:1353–4.

59. Campbell MJ, Machen D. *Medical Statistics: A Common Sense Approach.* Chichester, England: Wiley; 1990:7–8, 63.

60. Kassalow LM. Statistical and data management: collaboration in clinical research. In: Gaurino RA, ed. *New Drug Approval Process: The Global Challenge.* 3rd ed. New York: Marcel Dekker; 2000:289–310.

61. Bourgeois B, Leppik IE, Sackellares JC, et al. A double blind controlled trial in patients undergoing presurgical evaluation of partial seizures. *Neurology.* 1993; 43:693–6.

62. Davis CE. Secondary endpoints can be validly analyzed, even if the primary endpoint does not provide clear statistical significance. *Controlled Clin Trials.* 1997; 18:557–60.

63. Zipfel A, Grob P. How much detail on confirmatory statistics and exploratory statistics must a statistical report contain? *Drug Info J.* 1995; 29:479–82.

64. Cannon C. Clinical perspective on the use of composite endpoints. *Controlled Clin Trials.* 1997; 18:517–29.

65. O'Neill RT. Secondary endpoints cannot be validly analyzed if the primary endpoint does not demonstrate clear statistical significance. *Controlled Clin Trials.* 1997; 18:550–6.

66. Pocock SJ. Clinical trials with multiple outcomes: a statistical perspective on their design, analysis, and interpretation. *Controlled Clin Trials.* 1997; 18:530–45.

67. Lofters WS, Pater JL, Zee B, et al. Phase III double-blind comparison of dolasetron mesylate and ondansetron and an evaluation of the additive role of dexamethasone in the prevention of acute and delayed nausea and vomiting due to moderately emetogenic chemotherapy. *J Clin Oncol.* 1997; 15:2966–73.

68. Weintraub M. How to critically assess clinical drug trials. *Drug Ther.* 1982; July:131–48.

69. Franks P, Gleiner JA. The treatment of acute bronchitis with trimethoprim and sulfamethoxazole. *J Fam Prac.* 1984; 19:185–90.

# Methods:
# Patients and Research Setting

**3**

□

➤□ 6. Are the patients selected and enrolled in the trial appropriately?

➤□ 7. Are the inclusion and exclusion criteria used to select the trial patients appropriate, clear, and complete?

➤□ 8. How closely does the trial sample represent the type of patient who will be treated with the investigational drug?

➤□ 9. How similar are the trial drug therapy and regimen to that used in clinical practice?

□

An important aspect of a clinical drug trial is how the participants were selected and how representative they are of patients who will use the drug. The discussion of this process is usually located in the abstract and methods section of the article. The assessment of participant selection ultimately relates to external validity or generalizability of the findings. Poor extrapolation of the data often occurs because the healthcare practitioner fails to adequately consider differences between the trial participants and the patients who will actually receive the drug. Differences between these populations occur in age, race, concurrent diseases, or changes in end-organ functions (e.g., kidney or liver function). Dissimilarities occur in less obvious factors such as location or setting, patient willingness to participate, or drug therapy under research. These dissimilarities may be unavoidable or the direct result of biased or poorly arranged patient enrollment and management.[1–6]

Obtaining an appropriate trial sample is one of the many challenges facing the research team. A typical enrollment process is shown in Figure 3-1 and can be divided into four groups of patients. The first group is the research population and represents the pool of patients with the disease from which the trial sample is obtained. This group consists of all patients who seek care at the research location (or locations). Patients are then selected to participate in the trial if they agree and meet criteria used to include subjects (inclusion criteria) and do not possess any characteristic that would prevent them from participating (exclusion criteria). This group is called the eligible sample.

The trial participants are those eligible subjects who complete the whole trial. Patients who withdraw from the trial for any reason would not be included in this group. Finally, the target population consists of the patients in the practice setting who might receive the drug.[7,8]

**Figure 3-1** The Subject Selection and Enrollment Process

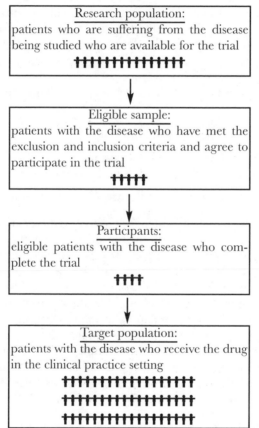

✝= Individual patients or groups of patients

As indicated in Figure 3-1, the number of patients available gradually decreases as more stringent participation requirements are instituted. The result is that a relatively small sample of subjects actually receives the drug, making the later estimates of the drug's effectiveness in the much larger and diverse target population difficult.[2,7,9]

This chapter addresses the complex challenge of identifying, enrolling, and maintaining patients needed to successfully generalize the trial results. The discussion focuses on how patients are selected (Questions 6 and 7) and how to compare their characteristics with the overall target population (Questions 8 and 9). Various problems are addressed, including investigator bias in the selection of participants.

# ☑ 6. Are the patients selected and enrolled in the trial appropriately?

The patient enrollment process selects subjects from the larger research population (Figure 3-1). Successful patient enrollment can be difficult and is dependent upon the type of medical condition studied and the size of the potential pool of patients. A properly designed clinical drug trial should always have a comprehensive process for enrolling subjects.[11-13]

The typical enrollment process begins when patients or their physician perceive a need for drug treatment. Patients may be enrolled in the clinical drug trial if[4]

- they meet the inclusion criteria,

- their physician is willing to participate and to abide by the clinical drug trial protocols and procedures, and

- the patient formally consents to be entered into the trial.

Once enrolled, the patient is assigned to a treatment group and must agree to assist or participate in the completion of all research forms. Because of the complexity of patient enrollment, investigators rarely report meeting their enrollment goals.[13-15]

When appraising the enrollment process, the reader must determine that the process resulted in similar study groups that were representative of the target population and that selection bias was minimal. Discussion of the enrollment process should indicate what method of selecting patients was used and the number of trial sites involved. In addition, if a trial objective is to examine the effect of the drug on a subset of the total sample (such as selected age groups), the method used to select the patients in the subset should be explained.[2,4,10-14]

## Selection Method

Study patients should be selected from the research population without bias or the data may not reflect the target population. The ideal method of selecting subjects is through random choice of patients from the pool of individuals who would likely receive the drug clinically. Random, in this case, does not imply that the sample is drawn haphazardly or in an unplanned fashion, but that each member of the trial population has an equal or known chance of being selected.[15]

Unfortunately, trial patients are rarely randomly chosen because of the unavailability of large pools of eligible individuals. The more common approach is to select eligible patients who either arrive consecutively at a research site or who are referred to the trial by a participating physician. This nonrandom enrollment process is sometimes called a "convenience" sample and is dependent on the bias or preferences of the individual who selects the patients.[2]

An important source of bias in a nonrandom enrollment process is the participating physician. In the treatment of cancer, for example, physician bias toward a particular drug treatment may be important in who gets selected for trials involving anticancer drugs. Reasons why physicians avoid certain patients were examined in a large, multicenter clinical drug trial on breast cancer. The most common reasons[16,17] were

- concern about negative effects on the doctor-patient relationship,

- difficulty with the informed consent procedure,

- uncertainty about investigational treatment, and

- conflict with the scientific requirements of the trial versus the clinical need to serve the patient.

Most patient enrollment and selection processes identify a group of patients based on a set of predetermined characteristics known as selection criteria. However, sometimes investigators are interested in studying the drug in a subgroup. The most appropriate approach is to create a group or "strata" where a specific factor (e.g., gender) is identified in advance and used to separate the eligible patient sample into subgroups. In this case, the study patients are selected and enrolled within each strata or group (*see* Chapter 8, Question 20). This approach is commonly called a "stratified random sample" if the selection method is random. If convenience sampling is used, the method is usually called stratified sampling.[18]

## Patients Who Are Excluded or Withdraw

Because published reports rarely describe the excluded patients, it is difficult to determine the number of potential participants eliminated during enrollment. The number is likely to be high based on the review[12] of 41 clinical drug trials, which indicated that only 34% achieved their projected enrollment figures, primarily due to patient or physician refusals. Hunninghake et al.[13] estimated that exclusion criteria and patient unwillingness to participate reduce the enrolled number to less than 10% of the expected number, particularly in large-scale multicenter clinical drug trials. Poor enrollment of eligible participants results in an over-representation in many clinical drug trials of Caucasians, married participants, and subjects with higher educational levels compared to nonparticipants (*see* Chapter 6, Question 17).[12,13,19–21]

One approach to excluded and withdrawn patients defines them as an "intention-to-treat" population. There are many definitions of this type of group, and the definition is dependent on the study design. The most common definition includes patients who entered the trial and received at least one dose of either the investigational drug or the control treatment. This approach is part of the Food and Drug Administration (FDA) guidelines for statistical analysis of NDAs. It is based on the concept that excluded or withdrawn patients may affect the results and should be considered in the analysis. Thus, the reader should review trial results carefully to determine if an intention-to-treat approach was included in the analysis.[22,23]

## ☑ 7. Are the inclusion and exclusion criteria used to select the trial patients appropriate, clear, and complete?

Existing information about the investigational drug is used to determine which patients receive the drug. This determination is based on inclusion and exclusion criteria. Both should be clearly written.[14]

Inclusion criteria give desirable patient characteristics for enrollment, while exclusion criteria involve characteristics that would prevent participation. Study inclusion and exclusion criteria must be clearly stated so readers can assess whether the patient selection process was unbiased. By using inclusion and exclusion criteria, investigators define their study population in a manner that is scientifically justifiable and desirable. In phase I trials, the potential risk entailed in administering a new drug to humans for the first time dictates that the trial group be relatively small and homogeneous. For phase III clinical trials, the selection criteria should be broader to approximate as closely as possible the type of patients who will take the drug routinely.[23]

In addition to clear inclusion and exclusion criteria to establish the generalizability of the results, information is needed to determine if the criteria intentionally or unintentionally introduce bias. Such bias would be the use of exclusion criteria to enroll only patients who would be most responsive to the drug therapy, e.g., treatment of excessively obese patients with an appetite suppressant drug. Another example would be including only the most compliant patients in a clinical drug trial testing the long-term effects of an antihypertensive.[6]

### Inclusion Criteria

Inclusion criteria are requirements that must be met by a patient to be eligible and are one of the most important parts of the trial design.

Inclusion criteria confirm that participants have the disease or condition under study and ensure that patients admitted are similar to those who eventually receive the drug clinically.[7]

The prerequisites for selecting patients vary significantly among clinical drug trials, primarily due to the differing backgrounds, experience, and philosophy of the investigators. However, they usually consist of demographic characteristics such as age, gender or race, medical condition, or other features such as medical setting and type of concurrent drug therapy allowed. These criteria should be expressed in clear, unambiguous terms and accurately stated.[24–26]

> **Criterion for age:** a precise age range for the participants should be established before the trial is initiated and should be consistent with the disease being investigated. It would be inadvisable, for example, to study an investigational drug for the use of migraine in patients under age 18, because the disease commonly occurs in older patients.
>
> **Criterion for gender:** the investigators should indicate whether only males, only females, or both sexes will be studied.
>
> **Criterion for medical condition:** a specific diagnosis or a diagnostic profile of a symptom cluster should be discussed and well established. The symptoms used to assess the patients need to be specifically described.

Inclusion criteria should be as broad as possible to ensure adequate patient enrollment and extrapolation, but narrow enough to exclude those who may be harmed or who are unlikely to benefit from the therapy.[24,27,28] Broad inclusion criteria

- simplify the screening process,
- increase the likelihood of meeting enrollment goals and obtaining a large sample size, and
- improve the applicability of the results.

However, narrower selection criteria are important because they

- increase the likelihood of achieving statistically meaningful results and
- enable the investigators to target patients most suitable for the investigated drug therapy.

One inclusion criterion often used improperly is the patient's willingness to participate. Enrolled patients should give every clinical and personal indication that they are willing to complete the full treatment.

Otherwise they should not be enrolled. A significant problem in clinical drug trials is that patients withdraw or are withdrawn because their obligations for participation were not clearly explained. The patient's right to withdraw at any time is always honored, but investigators must select patients who are likely to complete the study and avoid entering patients whose commitment is doubtful.[25]

While not really considered a selection criterion, the number of patients expected to complete the study is often included in the statements about the inclusion criteria. The expected total number of patients should be discussed, including any estimates of the number of patients who will withdraw or be withdrawn. If appropriate, the investigators should discuss any efforts to enroll larger numbers of patients to ensure sufficient numbers for meaningful statistical analyses.[25]

## Exclusion Criteria

Exclusion criteria are often not explicitly stated but describe characteristics that make a patient ineligible.[2] Excluded patients are those who

- are atypical of the population for whom the investigational drug was intended,

- are less likely to benefit from the therapy, or

- have confounding conditions (e.g., kidney disease) that make establishing drug efficacy and safety difficult.

The narrowing of the potential patient population by exclusion makes the trial groups more similar to each other and makes the assessment of differences between the investigational drug and the control drug easier. Unfortunately, it also reduces the extent to which the results can be extrapolated to clinical practice (*see* Chapter 9, Question 23). In addition, it is more difficult to recruit patients.[2,23,24,28]

Exclusion criteria should be stated clearly and explicitly. Any patient with a high probability of a drug nonresponse or who does not conclusively meet the inclusion criteria should be eliminated. Including patients with existing concurrent diseases that could compromise the investigational drug's efficacy should be avoided or at least restricted. Patients who may be allergic to the test drug should be excluded. The criteria should also exclude any patient whose medical history, physical condition, concomitant medications, or personal habits (e.g., smoking) might compromise the integrity of the data or might pose a safety concern. The reader must pay particular attention to the number of exclusions listed in the protocol; too many can make it extremely difficult to enter enough patients, and too few can lead to compromised trial results.[25]

Some typical exclusion criteria used in the past are currently being reexamined. For example, it was generally routine to exclude women of childbearing age because of potential risks and liability concerns relative to fetal exposure to drug therapy, despite the fact that many women practice birth control. Children and minorities were excluded because of concerns surrounding altered drug response or lack of availability of these patients for inclusion in drug trials. Patients from these groups are now included. The result is a broader range of clinical responses, including an increased probability that rare or difficult to detect adverse drug effects (ADEs) will be recognized.[29,30]

## ☑ 8. How closely does the trial sample represent the type of patient who will be treated with the investigational drug?

Regardless of the process, the individuals enrolled should be compared with the larger pool of patients (i.e., the target population) to determine how representative the reported trial results are (*see* Chapter 9, Question 23). The representativeness of a patient sample can be assessed by examining key characteristics of enrolled patients. Some key characteristics are listed in Table 3-1 and should be described in the article so that assessment of the similarity between the trial patients and the larger target is possible.[3]

**Table 3-1** Typical Sample Characteristics to Assess Representativeness

| Characteristic | Example |
| --- | --- |
| Patient demographics | age, gender |
| Medical condition | diagnosis, symptoms |
| Research setting | academic health centers, ambulatory settings |

### Patient Demographics

Historically, clinical drug trials primarily utilized young or middle aged white males. The results with such participants have limited applicability, particularly for certain age groups such as the elderly. Almost any drug effect in the elderly has greater variation than in the younger population, primarily due to differences in organ function, concurrent disease states, and concomitant drug therapy.[13,19–21,31,32] Women and minorities are two other groups often under-represented in clinical drug trials. Women were not represented in a National Institutes of Health (NIH) sponsored clinical drug trial on use of aspirin to prevent acute myocardial infarction, even though the disease is a major cause of death in women. The relatively low number of minority patients in NIH-sponsored cancer treatment trials may have produced misleading findings in types of cancer where race can influence the disease (e.g., cervical or esophageal cancer, myeloma). The problem of underrepresentation of women and minorities has led to NIH requirements that all submitted research proposals ensure gender and minority representation consistent with the known incidence/prevalence of the study disease.[19,33-35]

Recently, the FDA has become interested in testing drugs in what is considered "special populations": groups that have been historically neglected. These groups included children, women, and the elderly. Children were typically excluded from clinical drug trials until a drug had been safely evaluated in adults. Exceptions were if the drug was intended to treat a specific pediatric disease such as adult-onset asthma. The lack of drug testing in children was addressed in a 1994 FDA ruling that required the professional labeling for prescription drugs to include more complete information about use in the pediatric population. The lack of women in clinical drug trials resulted in a 1993 FDA recommendation that women of all ages be included in clinical trials and that results be analyzed by gender. The recommendation replaced a 1977 FDA policy that excluded women of childbearing potential because of the perceived risk of reproductive or developmental toxicity. The agency also encouraged drug sponsors to increase the number of older subjects in their clinical drug trials by publishing a 1997 recommendation that requires better prescription drug labeling about use in the elderly. Another FDA effort required that information about subjects enrolled in clinical drug trials show  important demographic subgroups (e.g., age group, gender, and race) and be included in all NDAs.[34-42]

## Medical Condition

The generalizability of the findings is limited if the investigator fails to clearly describe the diagnostic procedures used to identify the relevant medical condition. For example, in a review of 51 trials involving patients with congestive heart failure (CHF), only 23 (45%) specified criteria for the diagnosis of CHF. Even if described clearly, the standards used to diagnose major medical conditions may be ambiguous. The lack of standards creates inconsistency among patient outcome measures, causing difficulty in extrapolating the findings to clinical practice. This problem is illustrated in a review of the research on acute myocardial infarction. The diagnostic techniques used to detect acute myocardial damage have changed greatly since the mid-1960's as a result of the increased sensitivity of laboratory tests and more advanced autopsy techniques. The improved diagnostic process alone may have contributed to the significant decline reported in the rates of the disease from 1960 to 1990.[1,43,44]

In some diseases, the lack of a clear diagnosis is a function of a poor understanding of the disease, such as the enrollment of patients in clinical trials of drugs used to treat Alzheimer's disease. Because the only accepted diagnosis involves a postmortem neuropathological examination, definite establishment of the disease is impossible. Thus, patients are enrolled based on symptoms associated with dementia, which is often caused by Alzheimer's disease. However, other diseases, such as clinical depression, also cause dementia, and the use of this criterion may result in participants who are likely to be unresponsive to the specific drug therapy.[45]

Even if clear diagnostic criteria are used, the nature of the disease may affect the generalizability of the results. Clinical drug trials of diseases with variable courses (such as vasospastic angina, rheumatoid arthritis, CHF, and renal stones) may be difficult to extrapolate because participants are in different stages. A particular problem involves those patients enrolled during the most severe phase. Based on a statistical phenomenon known as "regression to the mean," such patients are likely to improve when measured a second time, even if other factors remain constant. Regression to the mean is defined as a set of unusual or rare values with a low probability of recurrence. Thus, any drug treatment appears to lessen disease activity, even though the change may be due to natural improvement.[46]

Although most clinical drug trials focus on enrolling patients with a diagnosed form of the target disease, some participants are entered into the trial based on their relatively better health, compared with the patients who suffer from the target disease. These individuals tend to be workers, volunteers, or personnel from organizations that typically encourage members to participate in drug research (e.g., the armed forces or the penal system). While healthy volunteers may be similar to the target populations, most are likely to not be completely representative. Even the use of healthy volunteers for drug toxicity studies can be misleading. In a trial of 398 healthy volunteers not receiving any medication, the investigators noted that 13% of the sample reported some symptom that could be attributed to an ADE. The most common symptoms were headache, coldlike signs, or backache.[32,47-49]

## Medical Setting

Many participants are recruited from academic research centers or hospital settings because these locations are more likely to include experienced investigators and are better able to skillfully handle new treatment procedures. Unfortunately, the patients who visit these settings tend to have advanced forms of the disease. Thus, these patients may respond differently to the test drug than individuals who typically use the drug clinically.[4,8]

Another factor to consider is the type of medical supervision. For example, a clinical drug trial involving a drug used to treat a chronic condition such as hypertension should be performed in an ambulatory setting similar to the environment in which the patient will be functioning.

The study should consider, and the article should discuss, compliance levels, an important problem with most drug treatments for chronic conditions.[50]

## ☑ 9. How similar are the trial drug therapy and regimen to that used in clinical practice?

The method in which drugs are used in a trial may vary significantly from their use in practice. [4,51,52] Differences may occur in

- how the drug is administered,
- the drug dose and schedule, and
- the duration of therapy.

To ensure that a suitable comparison can be made, a complete description of the drugs and how they are to be used in the study is needed.

### Administration

Articles reporting clinical drug trial results should describe how the drug was administered.[25,53] If appropriate, specific instructions such as mealtime dosing should be noted if their effects on drug dissolution and absorption rates or potential drug interactions are important. The route of administration in the clinical trial sometimes differs from what would be expected in practice. For example, drugs studied in the hospital setting may be administered intravenously to more severely ill patients, while in the ambulatory care setting the drugs may be administered orally or subcutaneously to less ill patients.

An example of the disparity between drug administration in a trial and in practice is pediatric use. If a drug is not approved for pediatric use, formulations are generally not available. This lack of approval typically means that a liquid dosage form is prepared extemporaneously, resulting in a potentially inconsistent product formulation for the child.[36]

### Drug Dose and Schedule

The dosage form of the investigational drug and the control treatments (i.e., placebo, capsules, tablets, injectables) should be described in all clinical drug trial articles. In addition, the strength of the study medication should be stated in milligrams, grams, grams per milliliter, etc. Daily minimum and maximum dosages should be consistent with the manufacturer's package insert or the dose range established during the early phases of clinical research. When appropriate, the actual dose schedule (e.g., daily, twice daily) and preferred dose times (e.g., morning and evening) should be provided.[25]

The dose and schedule used in many clinical drug trials often are based on the requirements of the drug development process. The amount and frequency are usually determined in phase I or II clinical drug trials (*see* Chapter 1) where the objective is to give the highest effective dose that will not cause serious side effects. These trials are sometimes called dose-ranging studies. Dose-ranging studies in phase I clinical trials are usually initiated very conservatively because little is known about the drug's effect in humans. The drug doses administered in phase II trials are based on the information received in the phase I trials and more closely resemble the dose range in clinical practice. The dosing protocols developed for phase III trials are based on the previous ranges and should be clearly established. If not, it often is an indication that the earlier phase I and II research was not adequately conducted. Higher doses are often required to avoid under-treatment or the ethical problem of administering subtherapeutic doses, especially for certain conditions such as severe infections. The dosing schedules used in drug development are sometimes too rigid and not based on uniform dose-ranging techniques. Thus, the total amount of the drug given during development may be too high for patients in clinical practice (resulting in increased toxicity) or too low (causing a suboptimal therapeutic effect).[25,51,54–56]

Part of the problem with establishing the appropriate dosing schedule relates to the limitations of the clinical development program and the overall drug approval process. While the goal of the program is to provide relevant information about the drug's safety and efficacy, dosing recommendations derived from this research are often inappropriate when individual dose adjustment is needed in practice. One reason for this limitation is that often only relatively limited data are available to model the pharmacokinetic and pharmacodynamic parameters and establish the proper dosing schedule. One solution is using what is called the "population approach."

Population pharmacokinetics is the study into the pharmacokinetic similarity and differences between individuals by measuring the drug level in patients who better represent the target population. This approach to establishing the proper dosing schedule is more effective than the traditional method of testing the drug in a relatively homogeneous patient population because it allows testing in a more diverse set of patients, such as those suffering from renal disease.[27,57,58]

## Duration of Therapy

Duration of therapy is important in assessing whether the investigational drug will be useful in practice. The length of time needed to establish clinical efficacy varies with the type of disease addressed. Drugs administered for the treatment of short-term conditions such as urinary tract infections are usually evaluated for a time period equivalent to the recommended duration of therapy in clinical practice. In these conditions, it would be inappropriate to continue treatment beyond the usual disease course. In contrast, the effect of tricyclic amine antidepressants takes at least 2–3 weeks to develop. Thus, patients should be observed for 3–6 months to judge the maximum efficacy of this type of medication.[4,23,25]

Unfortunately, determining an appropriate time period for the clinical evaluation of the investigational drug is difficult.[23,59] The many factors affecting the choice include

- the expense of performing long-term clinical drug trials,

- the regulatory requirements of the FDA, and

- the inherent methodological problem of measuring long-term clinical effects in premarketing clinical research (usually phase III).

The ideal timeframe would be long enough to administer the drug for the predetermined duration without dose-limiting side effects occurring, while still achieving maximum clinical efficacy.

The competing demands of getting a drug to market and the inherent limitations of the clinical research protocols in phase I–III trials result in varied interpretations of the accepted length. The variation can have negative consequences if the duration chosen is not suitable to thoroughly assess the drug's effects, particularly its safety. One approach to offset this limitation is through the utilization of thoughtfully designed phase IV clinical trials as well as overall increased monitoring (pharmacovigilance) of the drug through postmarketing surveillance programs.[2,59]

## Interacting Drugs

An additional concern in assessing the drug therapy of the trial patients is the presence of drugs in their regimen that may interact with the investigational or control drugs. While narrow inclusion and specific exclusion criteria can eliminate patients taking other medications, this approach is often impractical and significantly limits the generalizability of the trial results to clinical practice. Drug interactions for a new compound are generally unknown, so investigational drugs are typically introduced to patients in phase I and II research who are not taking concurrent medications. Once the investigational drug is used in phase III clinical drug trials, some attempt is made to compare the therapeutic and toxic effects of the new drug to patients both with and without concomitant drug therapy. If predictions can be made based on the compound's characteristics, drug interaction studies should be completed with medications that are more likely to interact with the compound. For example, a compound with high protein binding should be used with similar drugs that compete for those sites. However, like the identification of ADEs, the description of potential drug interactions with the investigational drug is limited due to study design and cost restrictions in most premarketing trials. A more effective approach is the use of phase IV trials to detect ADEs.[59,60]

Contraindicated medications should be listed in the description of the inclusion or exclusion criteria. The investigators need to ensure that only those drugs considered necessary for the patient's welfare are administered. These drugs should be comprehensively described, including their names, dose schedules, and duration of use. Clear guidelines should be given about the potential drug interactions considered.[25]

# References

1. Riegelman RK, Hirsch RP. *Studying a Study and Testing a Test.* 2nd ed. Boston: Little Brown; 1989:60–4, 147–9.

2. Friedman LM, Furberg CD, DeMets DL. *Fundamentals of Clinical Trials.* 2nd ed. Littleton, MA: PSG Publishing; 1985:23–30, 152.

3. Sackett DL. How to read clinical journals. I. Why to read them and how to start reading them critically. *CMA J.* 1981; 124:555–8.

4. Pocock SJ. *Clinical Trials: A Practical Approach.* New York: Wiley; 1983: 34–41; 66–8; 176–9.

5. O'Connell JB, Mason JW. The applicability of results of streamlined trials to clinical practice: the myocarditis treatment trial. *Stat Med.* 1990; 9:193–7.

6. DeMets D. Distinction between fraud, bias, errors, misunderstanding, and incompetence. *Controlled Clin Trials.* 1997; 18:637–50.

7. Elwood MJ. *Critical Appraisal of Epidemiological Studies and Clinical Trials.* New York: Oxford University Press; 1998:55–93.

8. Hansen EH, Launso L. Development, use and evaluation of drugs: the dominating technology in the health care system. *Soc Sci Med.* 1987; 25:65–73.

9. Campbell MJ, Machen D. *Medical Statistics: A Common Sense Approach.* Chichester, England: Wiley; 1990:54.

10. *Concepts and Strategies in New Drug Development.* Nwangku PU, ed. New York: Praeger; 1983:101.

11. Prout TE. Patient recruitment: other examples of recruitment problems and solutions. *Clin Pharmacol Ther.* 1979; 25:695–6.

12. Charlson ME, Horwitz RI. Applying results of randomized trials to clinical practice: impact of losses before randomization. *Br Med J.* 1984; 289:1281–4.

13. Hunninghake DB, Darby CA, Probstfield JL. Recruitment experience in clinical trials: Literature summary and annotated bibliography. *Controlled Clin Trials.* 1987; 8(suppl):6S–15S.

14. Berzon RA. Understanding and using health-related quality of life instruments within clinical research studies. In: Staquet MJ, Hays RD, Fayers PM, eds: *Quality of Life Assessment in Clinical Trials.* New York: Oxford University Press; 1998:3–15.

15. McAuley WJ. *Applied Research in Gerontology.* New York: Van Nostrand-Reinhold, 1987:130.

16. Ganz PA. Clinical trials: concerns of the patient and the public. *Cancer.* 1990; 65:2394–9.

17. Taylor KM, Margolese RG, Soskolne CL. Physicians' reasons for not entering eligible patients in a randomized clinical trial of surgery for breast cancer. *N Engl J Med.* 1984; 310:1363–7.

18. Elwood MJ. *Critical Appraisal of Epidemiological Studies and Clinical Trials.* New York: Oxford University Press; 1998:116–60.

19. Rehm D. Is there gender bias in drug testing? *FDA Consumer.* 1991; (April):9–13.

20. Svensson CK. Representation of American blacks in clinical trials of new drugs. *JAMA.* 1989; 261:263–5.

21. Kitler ME. The changing face of clinical trials. *J Hypertension.* 1988; 6(suppl 1):S73–S80.

22. Svensson K. How many populations must be analyzed and how should they be defined (intent-to-treat, eligible, per protocol population, etc.)? *Drug Info J.* 1995; 29(2):475–8.

23. Kassalow LM. Statistical and data management: collaboration in clinical research. In: Gaurino RA, ed. *New Drug Approval Process: The Global Challenge.* 3rd ed. New York: Marcel Dekker; 2000:289–310.

24. Yusuf S, Held P, Teo KK. Selection of patients for randomized controlled trials: implications of wide or narrow eligibility criteria. *Stat Med.* 1990; 9:73–86.

25. Gaurino RA. Clinical research protocols. In: Gaurino RA, ed. *New Drug Approval Process: The Global Challenge.* 3rd ed. New York: Marcel Dekker; 2000:219–46.

26. Subcutaneous Sumatriptan Study Group. Treatment of migraine attacks with sumatriptan. *N Engl J Med.* 1991; 325:316–21.

27. Aarons L. Pharmacokinetic and pharmacodynamic modeling in drug development (editorial). *Stat Methods Med Res.* 1999; 8:181–2.

28. Franks P. Clinical trials. *Fam Med.* 1988; 20:443–8.

29. Wilson JT. Questions and answers on labeling of drugs for children. *Drug Info J.* 1999; 33:375–83.

30. Van Der Laan JW, Olejiniczak K. Pharmaceutical testing and pregnancy: from testing to labeling. *Drug Info J.* 1999; 33:1125–33.

31. Bell JA, May FE, Stewart RB. Clinical research in the elderly: ethical and methodological considerations. *Drug Intell Clin Pharm.* 1987; 21:1002–7.

32. Svensson CK. Ethical considerations in the conduct of clinical pharmacokinetic studies. *Clin Pharmacokinet.* 1989; 17:217–22.

33. Friedman MA, Cain DF. National cancer institute sponsored cooperative clinical trials. *Cancer.* 1990; 65(suppl): 2376–82.

34. Anonymous. NIH/ADAMHA policy concerning inclusion of women in study populations. *NIH Guide.* 1990; 19:17–9.

35. Cockburn J, Redman S, Kricker A. Should women take part in clinical trials in breast cancer? Issues and some solutions. *J Clin Oncol.* 1998; 16(1): 354–62.

36. Nahata MC. Pediatric drug formulations: a rate-limiting step. *Drug Info J.* 1999; 33:393–6.

37. Hooymans PM, Janknegth R. Drug research in the elderly. In: Solgliero-Gilbert G, ed. *Drug Safety Assessment in Clinical Trials.* 3rd ed. New York: Marcel Dekker; 1993:83–91.

38. Merkatz RB, Temple R, Sobel S, et al. Inclusion of women in clinical trials—policies for population subgroups. *N Engl J Med.* 1993; 329:288–96.

39. FDA Center for Drug Evaluation and Research. *From Test Tube to Patient: Improving Health Through Human Drugs.* Rockville MD: Food and Drug Administration; 1999:18–23.

40. FDA Center for Drug Evaluation and Research. *From Test Tube to Patient: Improving Health Through Human Drugs.* Rockville MD: Food and Drug Administration; 1999:78–81.

41. FDA Center for Drug Evaluation and Research. *From Test Tube to Patient: Improving Health Through Human Drugs.* Rockville MD: Food and Drug Administration; 1999:82–7.

42. Alexander D. The pediatric pharmacology research unit network of the National Institute of Child Health and Human Development. *Drug Info J.* 1999; 33:385–91.

43. Marantz PR, Alderman MH, Tobin JN. Diagnostic heterogeneity in clinical trials for congestive heart failure. *Ann Intern Med.* 1988; 109:55–61.

44. Burke GL, Edlavitch SA, Crow RS. The effects of diagnostic criteria on trends in coronary heart disease morbidity: the Minnesota Heart Survey. *J Clin Epidemiol.* 1989; 42:17–24.

45. Gray JA. Clinical methodology of Alzheimer's disease trials. *Drug Info J.* 1999; 33:245–52.

46. Spector R, Park GD. Regression to the mean: a potential source of error in clinical pharmacological studies. *Drug Intell Clin Pharm.* 1985; 19:916–9.

47. Sterling TD, Weinkam JJ, Weinkam JL. The sick person effect. *J Clin Epidemiol.* 1990; 43:141–51.

48. Amori G, Lenox RH. Do volunteer subjects bias clinical trials? *J Clin Psychopharmacol.* 1989; 9:321–7.

49. Kulkarni RD, Vakil BJ. Baseline spontaneous symptoms in healthy persons—a prospective study. *J Clin Pharmacol.* 1975; 15:442–5.

50. Vrijens B, Goetghebeur E. The impact of compliance in pharmacokinetic studies. *Stat Methods Med Res.* 1999; 8:247–62.

51. Finkel M. In: Nwangku PU, ed. *Concepts and Strategies in New Drug Development.* New York: Praeger; 1983:17–22.

52. Weintraub M. How to critically assess clinical drug trials. *Drug Ther.* 1982;(July):131–48.

53. Bowden MI, Bion JF. Drug assessment in critical illness. In: Solgliero-Gilbert G, ed. *Drug Safety Assessment in Clinical Trials.* 3rd ed. New York: Marcel Dekker; 1993:93–110.

54. Polk RE, Hepler CD. Controversies in antimicrobial therapy: critical analysis of clinical trials. *Am J Hosp Pharm.* 1986; 43:630–40.

55. Sheiner LB, Beal SL, Sambol NC. Study designs for dose-ranging. *Clin Pharmacol Ther.* 1989; 46:63–77.

56. Chiou WL. Discrepancies in recommended dosage regimens of drugs. *J Clin Pharmacol.* 1976; 16:6–7.

57. Machado SG, Miller R, Hu C. A regulatory perspective on pharmacokinetic/pharmacodynamic modeling. *Stat Methods Med Res.* 1999; 8:217–45.

58. Sheiner L, Wakefield J. Population modeling in drug development. *Stat Methods Med Res.* 1999; 8:183–93.

59. Decoster G, Buyse M. Clinical research after drug approval: what is needed and what is not. *Drug Info J.* 1999; 33:627–34.

60. Kirby D. Adverse drug events in clinical trials. In: Solgliero-Gilbert G, ed. *Drug Safety Assessment in Clinical Trials.* 3rd ed. New York: Marcel Dekker; 1993:25–38.

# 4

# Methods:
# Use of Experimental Controls

❑

➤❑10.  Is the type of trial design used suitable?

➤❑11.  Are the appropriate control groups used?

➤❑12.  Is the patient assignment to the experimental and control groups randomized?

➤❑13.  Are adequate blinding techniques used?

❑

A primary focus of a clinical drug trial is to demonstrate that the test drug results in noticeable improvements in the condition of patients. This objective is usually accomplished by comparing the experience of one group of patients who receive the investigational drug (the experimental group) with a group of patients having the same condition who are not receiving identical drug treatment (the control group). Generally, if the condition of the experimental group improves relative to the control, the test drug is considered more efficacious, assuming that other potential causes are minimized.[1-3]

Potential causes could be chance occurrence, investigator bias, or the presence of confounding factors. The likelihood that the observed differences between the experimental and control groups are due to chance and thus are not true differences is termed chance occurrence. Chance occurrences can be addressed by repeating the experiment or managed by statistical analysis (*see* Chapter 8, Questions 20 and 21). The other factors, investigator bias and the presence of confounding factors, can be addressed by the study design.[4-7]

This chapter examines the approaches used by investigators to control confounding factors and investigator bias. Discussion includes a description of possible study designs (Question 10), type of controls (Question 11), different methods of assigning subjects (Question 12), and the use of blinding techniques (Question 13).

Often defined as a prejudice of partiality for a certain outcome (usually positive results), investigator bias may or may not be conscious. Thus, controls need to be instituted in a clinical drug trial to prevent successful guessing by the investigator, which may influence the interpretation of the drug's effectiveness.[5]

Confounding factors are events that affect the relationship between the test drug and the clinical outcome measures and may distort the interpretation of the results (*see* Chapter 9, Question 22). Numerous confounding factors can affect a clinical drug trial. One common factor is the possibility that the patient's illness may have simply run its course, and recovery would have occurred with no treatment. Another is that the patients in the experimental and control groups are substantially dissimilar from each other and thus respond differently to drug therapy. A third is that experimental and control groups receive different supportive treatment. A final factor is that the close similarity between the investigational and control drugs basically makes both groups similar in the care they receive. Investigators designing clinical trials must control as many of these extraneous factors as possible to ensure that the investigational drug is primarily responsible for the reported clinical effects.[1,3,4]

One limited method of control is the restriction of potential interfering factors through the use of narrow selection criteria. A more effective approach is the use of experimental and control groups. Their use is determined by the study design, with the most common approach being the parallel group design. This design involves two or more groups treated separately but concurrently as part of the same clinical drug trial.[8,9]

Another approach is the crossover design, which uses patients as their own controls; participants receive both the test and control treatments during separate and specified periods. A number of possible control groups can be used, depending on the drug being tested or the disease being studied. The most common control groups involve use of a placebo or an active control group. A less frequent approach is the use of historical controls in which the experimental group is compared to patients not enrolled in the present trial.[8,9]

Once the appropriate study design and control groups are selected, the investigator ensures that the groups are equal in everything except the administered drug treatment. The ideal method is the random assignment of patients to each group. The investigator must consider blinding techniques, which reduce the likelihood of investigator or patient bias toward a specific response.[1,2,10]

Most researchers believe that well-designed double-blind, controlled studies yield the most valid results about clinical drug efficacy. In fact, Food and Drug Administration (FDA) approval is often based on findings from a minimum of two double-blind, controlled clinical drug trials in which the test drug showed a difference compared to a control, usually a placebo. Although exceptions to this rule exist, such as fast-tracking drugs for AIDS treatment, the randomized controlled clinical trial is considered the most desirable approach. Results from uncontrolled trials should be considered as preliminary evidence and should rarely be the basis for clinical decisions unless the disease previously was uniformly fatal or if available treatments are ineffective or nonexistent.[6,11,12]

# ☑ 10. Is the type of trial design used suitable?

The design of a clinical drug trial organizes the experimental and control groups so that a fair comparison can be made. There are generally two basic types of trial designs: parallel (the most common) and crossover. More sophisticated derivations are the factorial and Latin-square designs.[13,14]

## Parallel Design

The parallel design compares the relative effects of different drugs or treatments on two or more groups treated separately but concurrently. Enrolled patients receive either the investigational drug or control treatment at roughly the same time. The basic design (Figure 4-1) involves two groups, although more could be included.[8,9,13,14]

**Figure 4-1** Parallel Design Involving Two Groups

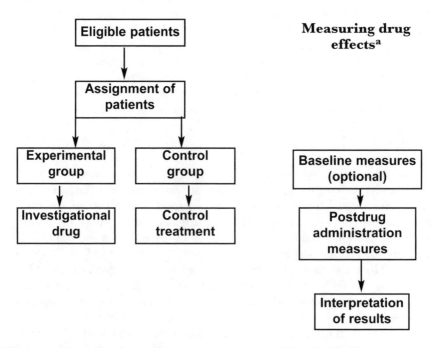

[a]Illustrates how the drug effects may be measured in this design

Advantages of the parallel design are that it is easy to conduct and may take less time to achieve the objectives. There is also a reduced potential for significant data loss because the patient is in the drug trial for a shorter period, and there are usually fewer measurements for each patient. Patients experience a potentially lower risk because exposure is limited to only one drug. A final advantage is that the more diverse set of patients and increased number of participants may increase the probability of detecting rare adverse drug events (ADEs). These advantages make the design suitable for phase I and II clinical trials because of its relative simplicity and low cost. An additional use would be in trials of drugs with long half-lives and high toxicity. Parallel designs are also suitable for longer term trials to minimize the effect of patient withdrawals.[6,14]

The major disadvantage of a parallel group design is the possibility of the experimental and control groups being different, although this disadvantage can be minimized with the random assignments of patients (*see* Question 12). The design also requires more patients than a crossover design and thus may be more expensive. In addition, the utility of the design is based on the assumption that drug responses from two individuals vary less than the drug response in the same individual, which is not true for all drugs.[6,14–16]

These disadvantages make the design less desirable for drug trials where random assignment of patients to the investigational or the control treatment is unethical or impractical. In these situations, a high probability exists that the study groups will be unequal. An example would be in the treatment of life-threatening diseases. Other examples would be the testing of drugs in diseases that are less defined or where drug therapy is not definitive. The parallel design is also not appropriate for most bioavailability or bioequivalence studies because it is less precise.

## Crossover Design

In drug research designs using crossover control groups, the same patient receives both the investigational and control treatment during separate, specified periods. The patient's reactions to each drug are compared to minimize the influence of individual patient characteristics on the response to treatment. As shown in Figure 4-2, patients in group 1 receive the investigational drug while the patients assigned to group 2 receive the control treatment. After an appropriate "washout" period, each patient receives the other drug, i.e., patients assigned to group 1 receive the control treatment, and the patients assigned to group 2 receive the test drug. This two-period crossover example is the most common and is referred to as a standard $2 \times 2$ crossover design. The key characteristic is that every patient receives both the investigational drug and the control treatment.[3,14,17]

The success of clinical drug trials using a crossover design is based on a control of various factors: carryover or period effects, treatment sequencing or drug order effects, and patient dropout or other data collection problems.

**Figure 4-2** Crossover Design with Two Periods and Two Groups

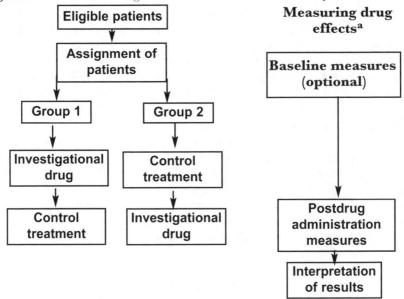

<sup>a</sup>Illustrates how the drug effects may be measured in this design

### *Carryover effects*

Carryover effects[6,13,18] occur when the pharmacologic effects of the first or preceding drug treatment persists during the administration of the second or subsequent drug treatment. The common approach to minimizing the influence of these effects is to delay administration of the second or next drug treatment by an appropriate period, which could be partially based on the drug's pharmacologic half-life (i.e., the amount of time it takes for 50% of the drug to be removed from the body). The time allowed for the delay of the next treatment is commonly called the washout period.

The washout period should be of sufficient length to allow for the effects of the first drug to be removed, approximately five half-lives. For example, the washout period for a study that compared the inhalant effects of the bronchodilators albuterol, isoetharine, and metaproterenol on airway obstruction in 60 adult men included a 24-hour washout period. This period was based on the knowledge that the half-lives of these drugs are less than five hours.[19]

In a crossover study, the drug-free and washout intervals must be defined and carefully noted. Washout periods should be observed before a baseline evaluation is made and before the investigational drug or control treatment is administered. Exceptions to the washout period conditions exist.

For example, if a patient exhibits symptoms of sufficient severity to warrant not withholding treatment, this patient may be entered into the study even though the washout period is less than that specified. However, the investigator should provide ample justification for including the patient in the analysis.

### Period effects

Period effects[6] appear when the condition under research becomes more severe, less severe, or fluctuates in severity during the trial. For example, drug treatment for a variable disease such as osteoarthritis would be difficult to evaluate using a crossover design because the fluctuations of the symptoms may mask the patient's response. Clinical drug trials containing large numbers of patients may reduce the effect of disease fluctuations because the variability of the disease would be spread evenly across the patients. Nevertheless, results reported from crossover studies with these types of conditions should be interpreted cautiously.

### Treatment sequencing or drug order effects

Treatment sequencing or drug order effects[6,14,16] occur when the sequence of drugs influences the results. An effective method to prevent such influences would be the random assignment of patients to the sequence in which each tested drug is administered. A rule should also be established prior to the trial indicating when the patients switch to the next drug treatment. The most accepted rule is to automatically switch at a set time. A less preferred rule is to switch based on how the condition is progressing.

An important advantage of a crossover design is that it minimizes variability in drug response because patients act as their own controls. Crossover trials also allow for more efficient use of patients (compared to the parallel design) because a smaller sample is usually required to compare the investigational drug to the control treatment.

The primary disadvantage of the crossover design is the length of time required for each patient to participate. Most patients would be involved about twice as long as patients in a parallel group design. This longer length results in problems such as the increased likelihood of patient withdrawal. The effects of patient dropout or other data collection problems are more pronounced using crossover control groups (compared with parallel control groups) because each patient represents a larger proportion of the data. Patient dropout rates can be high in crossover studies because patients must receive at least two treatments to provide enough meaningful information for analysis. Patient dropout and other data collection problems are less pronounced in crossover studies that involve short-term drug treatment with few severe side effects than in long-term clinical drug trials of more toxic drugs.

Another disadvantage is the increased exposure that each study participant may have to the toxic effects of the study drugs. Because the patient receives both the investigational drug and the control treatment, the likelihood of a severe ADE increases. This probability is especially high if the control treatment consists of an active drug or if either drug has a long half-life. The use of a placebo as the control treatment reduces the likelihood of a toxic reaction but increases the probability of allowing the disease to go untreated for an unnecessarily long time.

A final disadvantage is the possible overlap of the drug effects or significant variation in the studied disease. Interpretation of results is based on the assumption that the patient's medical and physical condition remains the same for the investigational drug and the control treatment. This is difficult to achieve, especially for the drugs with long half-lives and in clinical situations where the patient is taking other drugs. In addition, the severity of disease may vary from treatment to treatment.[14,16]

Crossover trials are only suitable if

- the effect is reversible,

- the treatment period is not too long,

- the condition is relatively stable, and

- carryover effects are not considered a problem.

Crossover trials are particularly advantageous if the within-subject variation is much smaller than that between subjects. That is, the drug response from the same individual varies less than the drug response from a comparison individual. This advantage makes it popular for studying the pharmacokinetics and pharmacodynamics of the test drug.[16]

In addition, such trials invariably require far fewer subjects than a parallel design and are less costly. Thus, the FDA recommends using the crossover design whenever appropriate in evaluating the pharmacokinetic and pharmacodynamic characteristics. The exceptions tend to be drugs with serious side effects or those used for progressive diseases (such as cancer).[6,14,16]

These designs should not be used in drug studies involving self-limiting diseases of short duration or with treatments that result in rapid relief or cures, because the illness may resolve and symptoms may be alleviated before the crossover takes place. Other drugs and diseases, such as narcotics for pain treatment, are appropriate to use with a crossover design as long as an adequate washout period is utilized and the pain is relatively constant.[6,14,16]

## Factorial Design

A sophisticated design used in clinical drug trials is the factorial design,[14,20,21] in which a several "factors" are examined simultaneously.

The factor is typically the investigational drug or the control treatment. These factors have "levels" that are the values or designations assigned to the factor. Levels in a clinical drug trial may be different doses or dose schedules, different combinations of drug therapy, or different lengths of therapy. The analysis is complicated and divided into "main effects" and possible "interaction effects."

The main effects are the changes in the patient's outcome induced through variation of the different factor levels. An example would be changes in patients' medical condition with different doses. The interaction effects are the joint effects of the drugs which are beyond the independent effects of each drug. If the drug effects are independent or have no relationship, there will be no interaction.

The primary advantage of a factorial design is that it allows the evaluation of the effects of multiple factors, both separately and in combination with each other. Parallel, crossover, and historical designs, in contrast, are limited to the evaluation of only one level or aspect. Factorial designs also offer economic advantages by reducing the number of subjects or observations needed. The number of factors and levels within each factor describes the dimensions of the factorial design. The simplest possible is 2 × 2. An example would be a study in which two drugs (i.e., the investigational and control drug) are compared at two different levels (with and without a placebo). A more complex version would be the 3 × 2 design, such as a study that focuses on assessing the effects of three different drugs at two different dose levels.

An example of a factorial design was reported by Lofters et al.[21]; the effects of dolasetron and ondansetron for the prevention of nausea and vomiting induced by chemotherapy were compared. The authors used a 2 × 2 factorial design to examine differences between two factors (types of drugs used) at two different levels (different combinations). The factors were the use of dolasetron, ondansetron, dexamethasone, or placebo. The levels were the different combinations: dolasetron plus placebo, dolasetron plus dexamethasone, ondansetron plus placebo, and so forth. The patients were divided into six research groups (Table 4-1).

**Table 4-1** Factorial Design for Comparing the Effects of Dolasetron and Ondansetron[21]

|         | Acute Phase (IV) First 24 Hr | Delayed Phase (PO) Days 2–7 |
|---------|------------------------------|------------------------------|
| **Group 1** | Dolasetron + placebo | Dolasetron + placebo |
| **Group 2** | Dolasetron + dexamethasone | Dexamethasone + placebo |
| **Group 3** | Dolasetron + dexamethasone | Dolasetron + dexamethasone |
| **Group 4** | Ondansetron + placebo | Ondansetron + placebo |
| **Group 5** | Ondansetron + dexamethasone | Ondansetron + dexamethasone |
| **Group 6** | Ondansetron + dexamethasone | Dexamethasone + placebo |

The primary comparison was between the effects of dolasetron versus ondansetron during the first 24 hours. Another comparison focused on the value of adding dexamethasone. Thus, the primary comparison involved group 1 versus group 4, while the secondary comparison involved groups 2 and 5 at 24 hours. In addition, the effect of the drug after 7 days was also examined.

In this study, the simultaneous comparison reduced the possible influence that changes in comorbidity, such as development of metastases to the GI tract or ascites, may have on the results. The disadvantages are that the design requires more patients (this study started with 703 patients) and may not adequately account for individual differences (especially important with subjective measurements of relief of nausea).

## Latin-Square Design

The Latin-square design is a crossover design in which the number of different drugs (or drug dosage schedules) equals the number of patients or blocks. The result is referred to as an $N \times N$ (e.g., $4 \times 4$) arrangement where $N$ is the number of treatments, patients, or groups. For example, a $5 \times 5$ Latin-square design was used to compare the hypnotic activity of five different drug treatments: single doses of flurazepam (15 mg), loprazolam (0.5, 1, and 2 mg), and placebo. The sequence of administration of the different drug treatments was randomized so that five groups of patients (12 in each group) received a single dose of one drug one night per week for five weeks. Although the actual sequence of administration was not published, a possible order is described in Table 4-2.[1,22,23]

**Table 4-2** Possible Latin-Square Design for the Study of Flurazepam and Loprazolam[23]

| | Group[a] | | | | |
|---|---|---|---|---|---|
| | **1** | **2** | **3** | **4** | **5** |
| **Week 1** | $L_{0.5}$ | $L_{1.0}$ | $L_{2.0}$ | F | P |
| **Week 2** | $L_{1.0}$ | $L_{0.5}$ | P | $L_{2.0}$ | F |
| **Week 3** | $L_{2.0}$ | F | $L_{0.5}$ | P | $L_{1.0}$ |
| **Week 4** | F | P | $L_{1.0}$ | $L_{0.5}$ | $L_{2.0}$ |
| **Week 5** | P | $L_{2.0}$ | F | $L_{1.0}$ | $L_{0.5}$ |

[a]F = flurazepam 15 mg; P = placebo; $L_{0.5}$ = loprazolam 0.5 mg; $L_{1.0}$ = loprazolam 1 mg; and $L_{2.0}$ = loprazolam 2 mg

An important advantage of the Latin-square design is that it can efficiently control against the influence of several factors (e.g., the sequence of administration and type of drug treatment used) while using relatively few patients. The major disadvantage is that it assumes that the factors do not "interact" (i.e., influence each other). The Latin-square design also requires a somewhat more complex randomization scheme.[24]

# ☑ 11. Are the appropriate control groups used?

The selection of the type of control groups is related to, but independent of, the design. The selection should be based on the information desired, ethical concerns, and the logistical challenges of the research. Control groups decrease factors that cause investigators to misconstrue results. Four frequently used types of controls are placebos, active or standard treatment, historical, or no treatment.[25]

## Placebo Controls

The placebo-controlled double-blind trial has been the gold standard in drug development for decades. It demonstrates the efficacy of a new drug in a confirmatory way by showing its superiority to placebo. The placebo control group uses the placebo alone or in combination with other types of control groups. In this type of control, the placebo is an inactive agent that resembles the investigational or active drug in all characteristics, such as appearance, route of administration, or dosage schedule.[25,26]

The purpose of giving the placebo is to correct for any psychological effects derived solely from medication taking or from receiving an injection. Participation in a clinical drug trial carries a nonspecific benefit with the patient responding positively to any intervention, whether it is the investigational drug or the control treatment. The placebo response is powerful, causing improvement in 30–80% of patients. These responses confound results and bias the assessment of the drug's efficacy. Thus, the use of placebo controls improves the likelihood that patients will not alter the reporting of symptoms to gratify their physicians or investigators.[26,27]

In addition, placebo controls minimize the influences of the investigator's natural partiality toward the positive effects of the test drug.[28] The value of placebo controls was demonstrated in a clinical drug trial of hypertension; some patients improved more on placebo, raising questions about the reported efficacy of the investigational drug.[29]

Placebo controls help investigators avoid the effect of confounding factors related to the natural history of the disease. For example, most acute and chronic pain problems are resolved whether treated or not. Illnesses such as endogenous depression and multiple sclerosis are characterized by cycles of remission followed by periods of active symptoms. Thus, the efficacy of the investigational drug may be incorrectly estimated depending upon at what stage the drug is introduced. Of particular concern would be treating patients who are at the extreme phase of their disease. The next stage is likely to be an improvement, regardless of whether a drug is administered. This tendency is known as "regression to the mean" and results in overly optimistic assessments of the efficacy of the test drug.[26,27]

An important use of placebo controls occurs in clinical drug trials of diseases in which no existing drug treatment exists. Here placebos help determine the specific value of the investigational drug, independent of other factors such as

- special attention by the medical staff,

- a positive physician–patient relationship, or

- the expectations of the patient.

An example of this approach is in the recent successful introduction of new drugs for the treatment of Alzheimer's disease.[28,29]

While placebo controls have advantages in establishing the true efficacy of an investigational drug, their use presents ethical problems and limitations when the findings are applied to practice. The ethical concern is that patients in the placebo control group are unfairly denied the benefits of drug treatment. Applying the results of a placebo-controlled trial to clinical practice is limited in conditions where acceptable drug therapy exists. Thus, information about the relative efficacy of the investigational drug would be lacking. Both issues are less important if no suitable drug therapy currently exists.[25,26,30,31]

## Active Controls

While the placebo-controlled clinical trial is the appropriate choice for demonstrating the efficacy of a test drug, there are instances in which the placebo drug may be unsatisfactory, e.g., when ample evidence indicates that existing drug therapy is effective. Thus, it may be more appropriate and ethical to establish that the test drug is not only efficacious but also superior to existing drug therapy.[25,31,32]

The control groups used for this objective are called "active controls" or "standard drug treatment." Use of active controls demonstrates that the investigational drug is superior or equivalent in efficacy and safety to the most commonly used drug therapy. An example would be the comparison of a new platelet antiaggregating agent, ticlopidine, with aspirin for the prevention of stroke. Sometimes the objective of using active controls is not to prove superiority but to establish that the test drug is equivalent. These types of trials are sometimes called "equivalence" trials. A fundamental purpose of such trials is to demonstrate that the test drug is not "inferior" to existing drug treatment, which implies that it is equally efficacious.[25,33]

The choice of the active control should be based on[6,25]

- the drug's relative efficacy,

- its safety profile,

- its ability to induce the placebo response,

- its acceptability in clinical practice, and

- the appropriateness of the dose schedule used.

Drugs that do not meet these criteria are used inappropriately as active controls. In the comparison of ticlopidine with aspirin for the prevention of stroke, the choice of aspirin as the standard was questionable because the drug had not been previously established to be unequivocally superior compared with placebo. Thus, although clinical drug trial results demonstrated that ticlopidine was equal in efficacy and safety to aspirin, it was not clear that either drug was very effective in preventing stroke.[33]

Active controls can be used instead of placebos or as a third group in a placebo-controlled study. Where it is unethical to deny treatment, the active control can be used with both groups and the investigational drug added to the regimen. In this kind of trial, all participants receive standard therapy approved for treating the disease, but those in the treatment group also get the investigational drug. The control group gets either no added treatment or placebo. Any difference in results between the treatment and control groups can be attributed to the investigational drug. An example is the phase III clinical drug trial that focused on the efficacy of paclitaxel for stage III and IV ovarian cancer. In this study, paclitaxel was used in combination with cyclophosphamide and compared to a standard treatment (cisplatin plus cyclophosphamide).[13,34]

## Historical Controls

Drug research designs using parallel control groups or crossover control groups are sometimes called "internal controls" because the patients are enrolled in the control group at about the same time as the patients in the experimental group. "Externally controlled" studies make use of control groups from another time period. These types of controls are also known as historical controls. Such controls use data from previously conducted trials or groups of patients treated earlier for comparison with the current study population. The comparison is based on an estimate of what would have happened without treatment. The historical control design is particularly useful when the treated disease has high and predictable death or illness rates. In these cases, investigators can be reasonably sure what would have happened without treatment.[10,13]

Historical control groups can be described or implied. Although some investigators report no control groups, they usually consider some comparison group even though it may be described vaguely as the "existing practice" of using a particular drug treatment or as "no drug treatment." Clinical drug trials using historical controls range from almost casual observations of possibly important relationships to tightly designed exploratory studies such as those used in phase I clinical drug trials.

Two common sources of historical controls are published external data or data already present within the organization. Published data consist of information collected from patients treated elsewhere but described in a publically available report. Such controls usually provide a poor comparison because it is likely that the experimental group is different from the control group in aspects other than drug treatment (e.g., patient selection procedure, experimental environment, and study measures).[1,35]

Data already present within the organization consist of patient information obtained from the same institution currently conducting the clinical drug trial, but during a previous period. Although more dependable than data obtained from outside the organization, reliability is limited because the reported analysis may be too vague to interpret, certain important factors or outcomes may not have been controlled or assessed, or some experimental conditions such as the type of patient tested were significantly different from the present research.[1,35]

Regardless of the source, the results from research using historical controls tend to exaggerate the effectiveness of a new drug treatment. In a review of similar treatments tested in which both randomized control and historical control designs were used, the trial results were different based on the type of control group. The new treatment was found effective in 84% of the trials that used historical controls, but in only 11% of the trials that used a randomized control design.[36]

Despite their limitations, historical controls are useful for rapidly obtaining initial impressions about a new drug treatment, particularly if the investigators emphasize the limitations involved in drawing conclusions or extrapolating the results. These impressions may be the basis for hypotheses to be verified by better designed clinical trials.

Historical controls are also useful in trials where there are significant ethical concerns regarding denial of the investigational drug to patients. An example would be the clinical drug trial that evaluated zidovudine (AZT) in patients with AIDS and advanced AIDS-related complex, where the progression of the disease without treatment would be rapid and deadly.[37]

When reviewing information obtained from clinical drug trials using historical controls, the reader should be skeptical about the value of the reported results. Nevertheless, the results can be useful if certain criteria are met.[10] The research should be directed toward

- an evaluation of the drug treatment for a specific disease similar to the one used in the historical control,

- specific objectives must be identified that are consistent with the current research, and

- clear differences must be established between the effect of the drug treatment in the present trial and the one used as the historical control.

## No Treatment[1,38]

Although ethical reasons make denying drug treatment difficult, control groups receiving no treatment or placebo should be used in clinical drug trials where effective drug treatment is not feasible or available. For example, a treatment group not receiving drug therapy would be useful in a trial evaluating the common cold. Because the symptoms of a cold are self-limiting, the investigational drug (e.g., a decongestant) should be compared with a control group that received no drug treatment. However, this type of control would be less useful if information about other possible drug treatments is desirable.

Controls consisting of no treatment are difficult to implement in patients unless adequate procedures are established to prevent the patients from taking unrecorded medications with effects similar to the test drug. These procedures include

- asking patients to report any additional drugs taken during the trial period,

- providing the control patients with a recorded number of medications to be used when needed to relieve severe symptoms, or

- institutionalizing the patient during the trial.

## ☑ 12. Is the patient assignment to the experimental and control groups randomized?

The method to assign patients to the experimental and control groups is usually described in the methods section and sometimes in the abstract. Discussion of this method is required by most journals and should include a clear description, including whether it was consistently used for all study sites (in the case of multicenter trials) and whether random assignment (the preferred method) was used. Regardless of whether randomization is used in the patient assignment process, baseline comparisons of the study groups should be reported. These comparisons should include important characteristics that may influence the trial results such as age, gender, race, medical condition, medical setting, or the presence of concurrent drug therapy.[6,9]

No matter how many groups the enrolled patients are assigned to, the assignment method must not introduce bias. In parallel designs, the experimental and control groups should be as comparable as possible. The most desirable approach is random assignment or allocation. A clinical drug trial that includes parallel control groups and random assignment of patients is called a randomized controlled trial (RCT) and is the most acceptable approach to allocating subjects.[1,3,9,24,29,36,39–41]

Random assignment means that patients have an equal and independent chance of receiving either the investigational drug or control treatment. Randomization diminishes patient and investigator bias by prohibiting investigators from assigning patients deliberately to a particular study group. By using nonrandomized assignment, physicians may place more seriously ill patients in the treatment group with the drug they believe to be most efficacious, thereby biasing the study. Alternatively, investigators may place healthier patients in the group receiving the test drug to demonstrate its superiority. With parallel designs, randomization is more likely than other assignment procedures to produce trial groups that possess comparable characteristics. These characteristics are sometimes referred to as baseline variables or covariates and should be evenly distributed or balanced between the groups. While randomization assigns treatments without bias, it does not necessarily produce balanced groups with respect to baseline characteristics.[3,9,24,25,39,42]

Ideally, investigators should describe exactly how patients were assigned and whether the process was successful. For parallel designs, investigators should begin the results section with comparative patient characteristics, including demographics, use of concurrent medication, and type, severity, and duration of the patient's medical condition. The investigators should briefly indicate (perhaps in tabular form) if the experimental and control patients are comparable and should discuss any statistically significant differences. When the experimental and control groups differ on known and important characteristics, their influence can be minimized by use of statistical techniques such as analysis of covariance (ANCOVA). ANCOVA adjusts for the baseline differences among the trial groups and essentially removes the influence of these differences from the analysis. While useful for randomized controlled trials, it is less effective in those trials in which patients are not randomly assigned. The baseline comparison is less important in crossover designs but should still be performed.[20,43,44]

Proper reporting of the randomization procedures should have the highest priority, and those trials that fail to provide such information should be interpreted cautiously. Reports of random assignment should include descriptions of[20,43,44]

- the type of randomization,

- the method of randomization sequence,

- how the assignment procedure was concealed from the investigators and the patient,

- who was responsible for executing the assignment scheme, and

- a comparison of baseline characteristics between the experimental and control groups.

Terms such as "random allocation" or "random trial" are appropriate in contrast to terms such as "without conscious bias," "systematic assignment," or "allocation at the investigator's discretion." It is also important for the reader to distinguish between the random "selection" of patients, which refers to the enrollment of trial participants, and random "assignment," which refers to the allocation of those already enrolled in the experimental and control groups.[42,45,46]

Although reports of clinical drug trials should demonstrate that adequate randomization occurred, this practice may not be as prevalent as expected. A comprehensive survey of the published research in the area of obstetrics and gynecology suggested that many authors were not very meticulous in publishing clear reports of the randomization process. A review of 206 trials in four major journals in the field indicated that 78% failed to provide information about randomization. In 11 reports (5%), the authors stated that the process was randomized but described a nonrandom process. Only 32% of the reports described an adequate method for generating random numbers, and the rates were similar among the four journals. Few reports stated who prepared the randomization scheme.[42]

## Types of Randomization Schemes

There are many approaches to the random assignment of patients to experimental and control groups. Some methods have a fixed or prespecified procedure (simple, blocked, and stratified randomizations), while other approaches adapt the random assignment process as the trial progresses (biased coin method).[1,39]

### Simple randomization

Simple randomization schemes[1,12,39,47,48] involve a prearranged sequence of random assignments in which each patient has an equal chance of being allocated to the experimental or control group. The advantage of simple randomization is that it is easy. The major disadvantage is a greater possibility that the baseline characteristics of the resultant experimental and control groups may be different, particularly if the sample or group size is small. In larger trials the statistical law of large numbers reduces the chance of serious imbalance, but smaller trials are more vulnerable to potential differences in baseline characteristics (*see* Chapter 8, Question 21). In fact, some researchers recommend that simple randomization schemes not be used in trials with a target of less than 200 patients.

An example of an important difference occurring between the experimental and control groups after simple randomization was noted in a clinical drug trial that compared indoprofen with pentazocine in the treatment of posttraumatic pain. Sixty patients suffering from pain due to fractures or serious sprains were randomly assigned to receive either the drug treatment or a placebo. Baseline measures were taken on self-assessment of pain severity (Table 4-3). The mean pretreatment pain assessment for the indoprofen group was higher despite the use of randomization. Because pain severity was the major outcome measured in this trial, the baseline differences among the groups could have affected results. Fortunately, the investigators minimized the baseline differences by using analysis of covariance.[48]

**Table 4-3** Baseline Self-Assessment of Pain Severity[48]

| Study Group | Pain Assessment[a] |
|---|---|
| Indoprofen | 3.45 |
| Pentazocine | 3.10 |
| Placebo | 3.10 |

[a]Average assessment of the severity of pain was made by the patient based on a scale of 0 to 4 with 0 = no pain, 1 = mild pain, 2 = moderate pain, 3 = severe pain, and 4 = unbearable pain.

One easy approach to adjusting for errors in simple random assignment is to repeat the procedure and replace the old assignment with the new one. This approach is known as replacement randomization and may be impractical in clinical drug trials that involve sequential enrollment of patients.[1]

### Blocked randomization

Blocked randomization[1,12,24,39] (also called permuted blocked randomization) is often used to offset imbalances in the trial groups by organizing the patients into numerical "blocks" such as four or eight individuals. The order in which the treatments are assigned in each block is randomized, and this process is repeated for consecutive blocks until all patients are assigned. For example, if the investigators want to ensure equality after every four individuals, blocks of four are created. The investigational drug assignment would be randomly arranged within each block as demonstrated in Table 4-4. As shown, the trial groups at the end of each block would be equal. Although baseline patient characteristics may be different initially, the groups should become more similar as the number of patients assigned increases.

**Table 4-4** Typical Assignment Sequence in a Randomized Block Design

| Block (four patients) | Sequence[a] |
|---|---|
| One | E-C-C-E |
| Two | C-C-E-E |
| Three | E-C-E-C |

[a]E = hypothetical random assignment to the experimental group; C = hypothetical random assignment to the control group.

Blocked randomization techniques are useful in clinical drug trials where the type or sources of patients recruited change during the entry period. This technique is also more likely to ensure balanced groups when premature termination of the trial occurs. A more common use of blocked randomization is the use of patients to study more than one objective. An example is the trial that examined the effectiveness of sumatriptan for migraine headaches. The primary study objective was to determine the efficacy and safety of sumatriptan in doses of 6 and 8 mg given subcutaneously. Thus, enrolled patients were assigned in blocks of six patients to one of three study groups: sumatriptan 6 mg, sumatriptan 8 mg, or placebo. Four patients in each block were assigned to the sumatriptan 6-mg group, while one patient within the block was assigned to the other groups. The purpose of the blocked randomization was to ensure that an adequate number of patients would be available to test the secondary study objective, which was to determine whether a 6-mg injection of sumatriptan after 60 minutes would benefit patients who did not respond adequately to the first 6-mg injection.[49]

A potential problem with blocked randomization occurs when the investigators know the size of the blocks. Thus, the assignment of the last person entered in each block would be known and could distort assignment. Solutions include using blinding techniques, avoiding blocks of two patients, or varying the blocking factor so that it is difficult to determine where blocks start and end.

### Stratified randomization

Stratified randomization[1,9,24,39,41,50,51] is another approach to problems with random assignment. It involves classifying patients according to one or more important factors (e.g., age, gender, race, medical setting, medical condition) before assignment. After classification, the patients are randomly assigned to the experimental or control group. To minimize the likelihood of producing dissimilar groups, this type of randomization should be used instead of simple randomization when the clinical drug trial consists of small sample sizes. In addition, stratification should be used in multicenter studies to ensure that the study groups are approximately the same size.

Stratified randomization is used to control for a factor that could interfere with interpretation of the results. The objective is to have the same proportion of patients from the different strata in each treatment group so that effective subgroup analysis can be done (*see* Chapter 8, Question 20). Whether the stratification process is simple or complex, comparability is the key.

This approach was illustrated in a clinical drug trial comparing benoxaprofen with ibuprofen in the treatment of osteoarthritis (knee or hip). In this trial, the investigators believed that older patients might react differently to the drugs than younger patients. In addition, they also believed that the location of the arthritis (i.e., knee or hip) might affect response. Thus, patients were stratified according to age (more or less than 60 years) and location of the osteoarthritic joint (knee or hip). Patients within each of these four groups were randomly assigned to receive either benoxaprofen or ibuprofen. Although no significant differences appeared when the age groups were analyzed separately, the benoxaprofen effect was more pronounced in the knee joint compared with the hip.

### Adaptive randomization

An alternative to using the fixed or prespecified randomization schemes is a method in which the assignment process changes as the trial progresses. This process is sometimes referred to as adaptive randomization[39,41] and includes the biased coin and urn methods of assignment. Biased coin assignment involves adjusting randomization so that the study group with the smallest number of patients will have a higher probability of having the next available study patient randomized to it. The major advantage of the biased coin method is that it protects against severe differences among the study group on key characteristics. The urn method of randomization is a type of biased coin design particularly useful with small sample sizes.

## Ethical Concerns

The most frequent objection to random assignment is based on ethical considerations. The typical argument is that randomization deprives half of the patients of receiving the benefits of the test drug. Critics have charged that physicians and other professionals engaged in clinical drug trials sacrifice the current interests of the patient participating in the trial to benefit all future similarly affected patients. Thus, random assignment would violate the personal obligation of physicians to use their best judgment and recommend the best treatment for patients, no matter how tentative or inconclusive the data on which that judgment is based.[37,52–54]

The ethical conflict has been magnified by the increasing number of patients with AIDS. These patients argue that the hopelessness of their situation should guarantee them access on a nonrandomized basis to drugs that offer some hope, even if randomized clinical trials have not been completed. Although such patients recognize that the investigational drugs are potentially toxic and may have limited effectiveness, some claim the right to take those risks.[37]

It is unethical for physicians and other healthcare professionals to engage knowingly in an activity that results in inferior patient treatment. However, the most ethical course is not as clear when the superiority of the test drug is not well established. The only reliable way to make this distinction in the face of incomplete information is to test the drug treatment using a randomized controlled clinical drug trial.[53]

The ethical problems of random assignment can be largely overcome if investigators adhere to a set of well-established guidelines. The generally accepted practice in the United States is that fully informed patients can consent to take part in a controlled, randomized clinical trial, even when effective therapy exists, so long as they are not denied therapy that could alter survival or prevent irreversible injury. The patients can voluntarily agree to accept temporary discomfort and other potential risks to help evaluate a new treatment. Thus, the patient needs to have a free choice whether or not to take part in the clinical drug trial. This choice is often referred to as informed consent. A data-monitoring mechanism also is needed so that the trial can be discontinued if a greater efficacy or toxicity of the test drug is clearly demonstrated.[37,53,54]

Additionally, the trial must be designed to have a definite chance of answering the question about the relative effectiveness and safety of the drug. This approach was used in the first clinical study of the AIDS drug zidovudine (AZT), when a clear survival advantage for patients who received the drug was observed relatively early. The trial was ended prematurely, and within a week FDA authorized a protocol allowing more than 4000 patients to receive zidovudine before it was approved for marketing.[13]

The most important justification for random assignment of patients to experimental or control groups is the existence of a scientific and medical consensus that the investigational drug has not yet been shown to be superior to standard or existing drug treatment. This principle is difficult to apply because of the tendency of physicians and other healthcare professionals to try newer drug treatments with the hope that their patients will benefit. Thus, random assignment should be done most often in the early phases of new drug investigations, when information is generally lacking about the relative superiority of the investigational drug and it cannot be plausibly argued that patients are at serious risk of being denied a more efficacious and safe drug treatment. An example of this approach occurred when the results of the National Institute of Health's Breast Cancer Prevention Trial, which enrolled more than 13,000 women at high risk for breast cancer, were announced. The preliminary results showed a 45% reduction in new cases of breast cancer in women who took the drug tamoxifen (Nolvadex) versus women who took a placebo. On the basis of the clear evidence of reduction in breast cancer in the tamoxifen group, those monitoring the trial recommended that the study be unblinded 14 months earlier than expected.[13,37,53,54]

## Nonrandom Assignment

While randomized assignment of patients is very desirable, some clinical drug trials involve nonrandomized assignment techniques. Nonrandom studies may show larger treatment effects than randomized studies and increase the risk of obtaining false-positive results. Thus, such studies must be viewed with caution. The healthcare practitioner who utilizes the results from a nonrandomized trial needs to determine whether the effects are so large that they are unlikely to be due to coincidence, design flaws (especially incomparable study groups), or investigator bias.[15]

Nonrandomized clinical drug trial reports should explain the assignment technique. Typical techniques are systematic or judgment assignment. The systematic method involves selecting and matching patients based on factors such as date of birth, date of appearance at the study site, or alternate numbers (i.e., odd/even). A version of the systematic approach is the assignment of pairs matched on the key factors described previously. Although systematic assignment reduces the possibility of biased allocation, it can be compromised if the investigator eliminates potential patients based on advanced awareness of what drug treatment the patient will receive.[1,24]

Judgment assignment is based on an assessment by the investigator or the patient's physician regarding the group to which the patient should be assigned. The major disadvantage of this approach is that the individual responsible for the assignment may consciously or subconsciously create significantly different experimental or control groups. Even when judgment assignment is based on "objective" assessments such as laboratory tests, it is impossible prior to the clinical drug trial to be aware of all important factors that may make the trial groups respond differently.[1,39]

Nonrandomized assignment of patients occurred in a trial comparing the effectiveness of cefaclor to that of amoxicillin in the treatment of urinary tract infections in a chronic disease hospital. The result of the assignment was groups of unequal size: 25 in the experimental and 36 in the control group. In addition, a comparison of the two groups of patients indicated a significant difference in the causative organisms of the urinary tract infection (Table 4-5). The presence of *Klebsiella* (resistant to amoxicillin) and a lower percentage of *E. coli* in the cefaclor group could have affected the response to the antibiotic and altered the comparability of the groups.[55]

**Table 4-5** Distribution of Causative Organisms by Study Group[55]

| Causative Organism | Cefaclor | Amoxicillin |
|---|---|---|
| *E. coli* | 53% | 79% |
| *Klebsiella* | 16% | 0% |
| *Proteus* | 13% | 17% |
| Enterococci | 8% | 4% |
| Miscellaneous | 10% | 0% |

# ☑ 13. Are adequate blinding techniques used?

The expectation of a positive outcome from the investigational drug influences patients' decisions to participate, resulting in the inclusion of a disproportionate number of patients likely to do well whatever their treatment. These same expectations may unintentionally bias the observations of both patients and investigators, either consciously or subconsciously. The result of this bias may be overreporting of positive results compared to negative findings. A specific bias to be addressed in the trial design would be the temptation to inaccurately record improvement in signs or symptoms attributed to treatment with the test drug. Clinical drug trials with such bias are likely to be ineffective in producing objective assessment of the test drug's efficacy. Along with random assignment, blinding of the participants could ensure that such bias does not distort the conduct of a study or the interpretation of its results.[13,56,57]

Although recommended for most trials, use of blinding techniques is particularly important in clinical drug trials in which the measures of drug efficacy are subjective (dependent on the impressions of the observers and the patients) rather than objective (based on quantitative assessments such as laboratory tests). Blinding techniques are also valuable for those trials in which knowledge of the drug used may affect the way the results are interpreted or the manner in which care is administered.[3]

## Investigator Bias

Even the most well-intended investigator can inadvertently interpret trial results consistent with pretrial personal interests.[3,37] The opposite effect also occurs: the investigator overcompensates for potential biases by interpreting positive drug effects negatively. The potential for bias increases as the involvement of the investigator in the measurement process increases (e.g., assessment of pain, the severity of possible side effects, or improvement in moods).

Although all aspects of the clinical drug trial should be protected against investigator bias, achieving this goal may not always be possible. Masking the drug effect would be very difficult in trials in which one or more of the drug actions is well known. This problem was illustrated in a trial of the effects of the cardiovascular drug propranolol in reducing mortality of postmyocardial infarction patients. Physicians were able to guess whether the patient was taking the drug or placebo approximately 60% of the time because of their knowledge of the pharmacological effects of propranolol.[56]

## Patient Bias

Biased patient response[3,27,46,56–59] to an investigational drug is commonly called the placebo effect. The placebo effect usually involves a patient telling investigators what they want to hear. Placebo effects may mask or distort the actual drug effects. Almost every patient–investigator encounter has a symbolic dimension that could produce a placebo effect. In fact, the placebo response does not require a placebo. The desired success of the treatment can be felt so strongly by one or both of the parties involved that objectivity cannot be guaranteed.

In addition, the act of giving a drug treatment can be a strong stimulus in itself. Thus, it is not surprising that placebos alter virtually any disease that can be reversed. The placebo effect involves a wide variety of responses, ranging from "subjective" responses such as mood changes to "objective" responses such as the spontaneous disappearance of warts. Biological/disease processes affected by the placebo effect include:[46]

| | | |
|---|---|---|
| Fever | Postoperative pain | Headache |
| Blood cell count | Cough reflex | Vasomotor function |
| Common cold | Adrenal gland function | Insomnia |
| Gastric secretion/motility | Mood changes | Blood pressure |
| Angina | Respiratory rates | Warts |
| Pupil movement | | |

The confounding effect of the placebo response on the findings of clinical drug trials is well documented. Some investigators estimate that about one-third of patients display a placebo effect in response to drug treatment, although much higher rates have been observed. Predicting who will exhibit this behavior is difficult because of the lack of agreement on what constitutes a placebo effect.[3,27,46,56-59]

The placebo effect can be influenced by the drugs being compared. Patients are more likely to identify a placebo if the investigational drug has prominent therapeutic or toxic effects. In a trial of this phenomenon, patients were asked to guess whether they received a placebo or phenyl-propanolamine, a drug used as an adjunct for weight control. While the effect of phenylpropanolamine on appetite suppression is modest, the drug has prominent side effects such as dry mouth and heart palpitations. Based on the prominence of these side effects, 75% of the patients receiving the placebo correctly guessed their treatment compared to only 43% of the patients receiving phenylpropanolamine.[60]

When the drug side effects are not as prominent, patients have a tendency to believe they are receiving the investigational drug rather than the placebo. In a trial of the effects of the cardiovascular drug propranolol (which has a low incidence of side effects), patients taking the drug were more likely to guess correctly (64%) than those taking the placebo (41%).[56]

## Blinding Techniques[3,6,25,26,57,60,61]

Protection against patient or investigator bias is accomplished by using single-blind and double-blind designs. Usually in a single-blind trial, the investigator, but not the patient, is aware of the treatment. A less frequent variation would be for the investigator, but not the patient, to be unaware of what drug is being given. In a double-blind trial, neither the patient nor the investigator is aware of which treatment the patient has received until the code is broken or the results are ready to be analyzed. A derivation of the double-blind technique occurs when both patients and investigators are unaware of assignment of subjects to experimental or control groups and a third group, which is responsible for the interpretation of data, is also unaware of the patient's assignment status to the experimental or control group. This approach is sometimes referred to as a "triple-blind" trial, although more commonly still considered a double-blind study.

The placebo-controlled double-blind trial has been the gold standard in drug development for many decades. It demonstrates the efficacy of a test drug by showing its superiority to placebo using relatively unbiased techniques to measure drug response. The double-blind design is usually accomplished by giving a placebo (which could be an active drug or inert substance) to the control group that is made to look, taste, and smell like the investigational drug, so that both the investigator and patient are masked from identifying the actual treatment.

In published research papers, the investigator should describe the blinding techniques comprehensively. This information should provide a complete description of the medication, including the form of the drug and placebo (i.e., capsules, tablets, injectables). A description of the methods of preparing the drugs (for example, the use of lactose or sucrose fillers) would be desirable, especially for the placebo, as well as the way the study drugs (investigational and active control) will be blinded. If an active control drug is used, information about the drug that exists in the product labeling should be included. The dose and dosage form of each drug must be listed (e.g., "capsules containing 10 mg of drug X").

The proper labeling of all medications is important during a clinical trial, and it is essential that the blinding of the study drugs be protected. For example, the labels containing the code of study drugs should be designed so that no member of the research team is aware of which medication is being administered or dispensed. The sealed labels contain decoding information opened only in the event of an emergency or an adverse experience necessitating drug identification.

Drug code labels come in many forms. One of the most reliable is the dual-label form, in which the code is covered by a mercury film that can be removed quickly to reveal the drug identity. Another effective type is the three-sided envelope with a detached section containing the written code. If an emergency arises, the detached code label portion is immersed in water for 2 minutes and then peeled apart. If not used for emergency purposes, the coded portion should be removed prior to dispensing the medication and returned to the sponsor at the study conclusion. This method determines the extent to which protocol deviations occurred (*see* Chapter 6, Question 16).

Pharmaceutical manufacturers usually supply their products, placebo, and comparison drugs in identical forms for most clinical drug trials. However, such an approach may be ineffective if the investigational drug and the active control drug have dissimilar formulations, such as tablets versus syrups, ampules versus suppositories, or liquid concentrates versus capsules. Additional blinding problems are presented by variations in physical characteristics, including color, taste, texture, viscosity, shape, or size. If a study calls for the comparison of two drugs with formulations that make physical matching impossible, the problem can be solved by the double-placebo (double-dummy) method. It consists of simultaneously administering to each patient an active test agent and a placebo of the other active agent being evaluated.

An example of the double-dummy method would be the comparison of an investigational drug present in only liquid form with an active control drug present in only tablet form. Two formulations would be given to each patient at each dose time. Patients in the experimental group would receive the investigational drug in liquid form and a placebo as a tablet. Patients in the control group would receive the active drug control in tablet form and a placebo as a liquid. Because the two formulations are administered simultaneously to each patient at all times during the trial, it would be difficult to distinguish the difference between active drug and placebo.

The procedure also can accommodate the double-blind evaluation of two active agents that must be administered at different times of the day because of their dissimilar modes of action. An example would be a comparison between an investigational drug (in tablet form) administered once daily (in the morning) and an active control drug (in capsule form) administered twice a day (morning and evening). The investigational drug plus a placebo could be administered in the morning to patients in the experimental group and two placebos could be administered in the evening. The active control drug plus placebo could be administered in the morning and in the evening.

Investigators generally indicate when they have used blinding techniques in the clinical drug trial. The absence of any reference to these techniques in the description of the trial design should be sufficient evidence that blinding methods were not used. In addition, the reader should be wary of vague or misleading terms when investigators indicate whether blinding techniques were used. An example is the use of the term "open label," which generally means that both the investigator and the patient were aware of the drugs used. However, the term may not be widely known in practice and could mislead the reader unfamiliar with the expression.

Few investigators report the success or failure of their blinding techniques. One cause of failure is the accidental breaking of the code, which should not occur in an adequately managed clinical drug trial. The only justification for prematurely breaking the blinding code is when a patient has an adverse reaction that necessitates knowing which treatment the patient received. The method of labeling the study drugs should allow this identification to occur without revealing the randomization code for the entire study. One such technique is for each medication container to have a two-part label, one of which is a sealed, tear-off section containing the drug identity. At the time the patient begins treatment, the tear-off section is detached and affixed to the patient's case report form to be opened in an emergency.

Problems with blinding are more prominent when single-blind methods are used because of the greater likelihood of an informed participant (e.g., a member of the research staff) revealing critical information about the design to the patient. Blinding techniques are usually desirable in clinical drug trials for the treatment of conditions in which spontaneous variation or remission is common (e.g., rheumatoid arthritis, ulcerative colitis, angina, or peptic ulcer disease). The techniques are also more likely to be effective when indirect measures such as laboratory tests or X-rays are used. These measures are less likely to reveal the identity of the drug treatment. No matter how rigorous the enforcement of blinding techniques, circumstances may arise that threaten the integrity of the blindness. For example, a larger number of adverse reactions in one treatment group compared with another may provide a clue about which treatment is involved, particularly in placebo-controlled studies. In addition, different patterns of symptom response in treatment groups may make identification of the investigational drug easier.

## Nonblinding Techniques (Open-Label Trials)

Nonblinding techniques, commonly called open-label trials, are needed when blinded studies are impractical or unethical. An example would be a clinical trial in which an investigational drug therapy is compared to surgical procedures or when certain drug characteristics (e.g., side effects, physicochemical properties, taste, and smell) allow easy detection of active versus control drug.[6]

Open-label trials sometimes extend the amount of information collected from a double-blind, placebo-controlled study. In these studies, typically phase III trials, an open-label phase is included to acquire more safety data about the test drug. The rationale here is that the clinical efficacy of an investigational drug may be established in relatively less time with fewer patients than can its safety, especially for relatively rare and unpredictable ADEs.[6]

Additional clinical efficacy information is sometimes collected in the open-label phase when the test drug is used to treat chronic medical conditions. Another use of the open-label phase of a double-blind trial is to compensate patients from the control group for participating in the trial by offering them the opportunity to receive the investigational drug after the initial study phase is completed. An example of both approaches occurred in the large-scale trial of tamoxifen for the prevention of breast cancer in high-risk women.[13]

While useful as a measure of drug safety, open-label studies have limited value in examining drug efficacy. The likelihood of bias is higher than in blinded studies, although this problem could be partially addressed by using outside evaluators unaware of the treatments to analyze the data. Nevertheless, the results of open-label clinical drug trials should be viewed with caution and should only have a limited influence on the use of the investigational drug in practice.[13]

# References

1. Pocock SJ. *Clinical Trials: A Practical Approach.* New York: Wiley, 1983: 4,50–90.

2. Polk RE, Hepler CD. Controversies in antimicrobial therapy: critical analysis of clinical trials. *Am J Hosp Pharm.* 1986; 43:630–40.

3. Cuddy PG, Elenbaas RM, Elenbaas JK. Evaluating the medical literature. Part I: abstract, introduction, methods. *Ann Emerg Med.* 1983;12:549–55.

4. Elwood MJ. *Critical Appraisal of Epidemiological Studies and Clinical Trials.* New York: Oxford University Press; 1998:116–60.

5. DeMets D. Distinction between fraud, bias, errors, misunderstanding, and incompetence. *Controlled Clin Trials.* 1997; 18:637–50.

6. Gaurino RA. Clinical research protocols. In: Gaurino RA, ed. *New Drug Approval Process: The Global Challenge.* 3rd ed. New York: Marcel Dekker; 2000:219–46.

7. Guyatt G, Sackett D, Taylor DW, et al. Determining optimal therapy-randomized trials in individual patients. *N Engl J Med.* 1986; 314:889–92.

8. Campbell MJ, Machin D. *Medical Statistics: A Common Sense Approach.* New York: Wiley, 1990:5–13.

9. Lavori PW, Louis TA, Bailar JC, et al. Designs for experiments-parallel comparisons of treatment. *N Engl J Med.* 1983; 309:1291–8.

10. Bailar JC, Louis TA, Lavori PW, et al. Statistics in practice: studies without internal controls. *N Engl J Med.* 1984; 311:156–62.

11. FDA Center for Drug Evaluation and Research. *From Test Tube to Patient: Improving Health Through Human Drugs.* Rockville MD: Food and Drug Administration; 1999:29–32.

12. Ioannides JP, Cappelleri JC, Sacks HS, et al. The relationship between study design, results, and reporting of randomized clinical trials of HIV infection. *Controlled Clin Trials.* 1997; 18:431–44.

13. FDA Center for Drug Evaluation and Research. *From Test Tube to Patient: Improving Health Through Human Drugs.* Rockville MD: Food and Drug Administration; 1999:18–23.

14. DeMuth JE; *Basic Statistics and Pharmaceutical Statistical Applications.* New York: Marcel Dekker; 1999.

15. McKee M, Britton A, Black N, et al. Methods in health services research: interpreting evidence: choosing between randomized and non-randomized studies. *Br Med J.* 1999; 8:312–5.

16. Senn S, Ezzet F. Clinical cross-over trials in phase I. *Stat Methods Med Res.* 1999; 8:263–78.

17. Louis TA, Lavori PW, Bailar JC, et al. Crossover and self-controlled designs in clinical research. *N Engl J Med.* 1984; 310:24–31.

18. Berezuk GP, Schondelmeyer SW, Seidenfeld JJ, et al. Clinical comparison of albuterol, isoetharine, and metaproterenol given by aerosol inhalation. *Clin Pharm.* 1983; 2:129–34.

19. United States Pharmacopeia. *Drug Information for the Health Professional.* 20th ed. Rockville MD: United States Pharmacopeial Convention, Inc., 2000

20. Bolton S. *Pharmaceutical Statistics: Practical and Clinical Applications.* New York: Marcel Dekker; 1990.

21. Lofters WS, Pater JL, Zee B, et al. Phase III double-blind comparison of dolasetron mesylate and ondansetron and an evaluation of the additive role of dexamethasone in the prevention of acute and delayed nausea and vomiting due to moderately emetogenic chemotherapy. *J Clin Oncol.* 1997; 15:2966–73

22. Neter J, Wasserman W, Kutner MH. *Applied Linear Statistical Models.* Boston: RD Irwin; 1990: 1083–8.

23. Elie R, Caille G, Levasseur FA, et al.Comparative hypnotic activity of single doses of loprazolam, flurazepam, and placebo. *J Clin Pharmacol.* 1983; 23:32–6.

24. Hallstrom A, Davis K. Imbalance in treatment assignments in stratified blocked randomization. *Controlled Clin Trials.* 1988; 9:375–82.

25. Hwang I, Morikawa Toshihiko. Design issues in noninferiority/equivalence trials. *Drug Info J.* 1999; 33:1205–18.

26. Lyons DJ. Use and abuse of placebo in clinical trials. *Drug Info J.* 1999; 33:261–4.

27. Turner J, Deyo RA, Loesser J, et al. The importance of placebo effects in pain treatment and research. *JAMA.* 1994; 271(20):1609–14.

28. Ritter JM. Placebo-controlled,double blind clinical trials can impede medical progress. *Lancet.* 1980; 1:1126–7.

29. Kitler ME. The changing face of clinical trials. *J Hypertension.* 1988; 6(suppl 1):S73–S80.

30. Brody B. When are placebo-controlled trials no longer applicable. *Controlled Clin Trials.* 1997; 18:602–12.

31. Temple RJ. When are clinical trials of a given agent vs. placebo no longer appropriate or feasible. *Controlled Clin Trials.* 1997; 18:613–20.

32. Lewis MA, Fishman DA. Ondansetron for postoperative nausea and vomiting: decisions in the absence of comparative trials. *Am J Health Sys Pharm.* 1994; 51:524–5.

33. MaKuch R, Johnson M. Issues in planning and interpreting active control equivalence studies. *J Clin Epidemiol.* 1989; 42:503–11.

34. McGuire WP, Hoskins WJ, Brady MF, et al. Cyclophosphamide and cisplatin compared with paclitaxel and cisplatin in patients with stage III and stage IV ovarian cancer. *N Engl J Med.* 1996; 334:1–6.

35. Einarson TR, McGhan WF, Bootman JL, et al. Meta-analysis: quantitative integration of independent research results. *Am J Hosp Pharm.* 1985; 42:1957–64.

36. Inglefinger FJ. The randomized clinical trial. *N Engl J Med.* 1972; 287:100–1.

37. Veatch RM. Drug research in humans: the ethics of nonrandomized access. *Clin Pharm.* 1989; 8:366–70.

38. Gehlbach SH. *Interpreting the Medical Literature: A Clinician's Guide.* New York, Macmillan; 1988:70–4.

39. Friedman LM, Furberg CD, DeMets DL. *Fundamentals of Clinical Trials.* 2nd ed. Littleton, MA: PSG Publishing; 1985:34–65.

40. Sacks H, Chalmers TC, Smith H. Sensitivity and specificity of clinical trials: randomized versus historical controls. *Arch Intern Med.* 1983; 143:753–5.

41. Kassalow LM. Statistical and data management: collaboration in clinical research. In: Gaurino RA, ed. *New Drug Approval Process: The Global Challenge.* 3rd ed. New York: Marcel Dekker; 2000:289–310.

42. Schulz KF, Chalmers I, Grimes DA, et al. Assessing the quality of randomization from reports of controlled trials published in obstetrics and gynecology journals. *JAMA.* 272; 2:125–8.

43. Koch GG, Tangen CM. Nonparametric analysis of covariance and its role in noninferiority clinical trials. *Drug Info J.* 1999; 33:1145–59.

44. Rochon J. Issues in adjusting for covariates arising postrandomization in clinical trials. *Drug Info J.* 1999; 33:1219–28.

45. Sackett DL. How to read clinical journals: I. Why to read them and how to start reading them critically. *CMA J.* 1981; 124:555–8.

46. Mosteller F, Gilbert JP, McPeek B. Reporting standards and research strategies for controlled trials. *Controlled Clin Trials.* 1980; 1:37–58.

47. Wei LJ, Lachin JM. Properties of the urn randomization in clinical trials. *Controlled Clin Trials.* 1988; 9:345–64.

48. Soave G, Lavezzari M, Ferrati G, et al. Indoprofen and pentazocine in post-traumatic pain. A double-blind, parallel-group comparative trial. *J Int Med Res.* 1983; 11:354–7.

49. Subcutaneous Sumatriptan Study Group. Treatment of migraine attacks with sumatriptan. *N Engl J Med.* 1991; 325:316–21.

50. Lachin JM. Statistical properties of randomization in clinical trials. *Controlled Clin Trials.* 1988; 9:289–311.

51. Tyson VCH, Gynne A. A comparative trial of benoxaprofen and ibuprofen in osteoarthritis in general practice. *J Rheumatol.* 1980; 7(suppl 6):132–8.

52. Hellman S, Hellman DS. Of mice but not men: problems of the randomized clinical trial. *N Engl J Med.* 1991; 324:1585–9.

53. Passamani E. Clinical trials-are they ethical? *N Engl J Med.* 1991; 324:1589–92.

54. Kodish E. Ethical considerations in randomized controlled clinical trials. *Cancer.* 1990; 65:2400–4.

55. Lindon R. Comparison of cefaclor and amoxicillin in the treatment of urinary infections in a chronic disease hospital. *Postgraduate Med.* 1979; 55(suppl 4):67–9.

56. Byington RP, Curb JD, Mattson ME. Assessment of double-blindness at the conclusion of the beta blocker heart attack trial. *JAMA.* 1985; 253:1733–6.

57. Ederer F. Patient bias, investigator bias, and the double-masked procedure in clinical trials. *Am J Med.* 1975; 58:295–9.

58. Bush PJ. The placebo effect. *J Am Pharm Assoc.* 1974; NS14:671–4.

59. Brody H. The placebo response (Parts I-II). *Drug Ther.* 1986 (July):106, 115–22,131.

60. Moscucci M, Byrne L, Weintraub M, et al. Blinding, unblinding, and the placebo effect: an analysis of patients' guesses of treatment assignment in a double-blind clinical trial. *Clin Pharmacol Ther.* 1987; 41:259–65.

61. Elwood MJ. *Critical Appraisal of Epidemiological Studies and Clinical Trials.* New York: Oxford University Press; 1998:55–93.

# Methods: Measurement of Results

□

> □ 14. Are the drug outcome measures clearly described and suitable?

> □ 15. Is the system of measuring the drug outcomes appropriate and adequately described?

□

An important feature of a clinical drug trial is how the desired outcomes are measured. The measurement system is usually discussed in the methods section of the article and includes a plan to collect comprehensive, systematic, and nonbiased data about the drug effects. The key is the measures used. These measures assess the investigational drug relative to clinical efficacy, safety, quality of life, and economic costs. After the data are collected, a system to organize and interpret the data is needed.

From a regulatory perspective, the objective of the measurement system is to provide enough data to convince Food and Drug Administration (FDA) officials of safety and efficacy by using the methods that FDA statisticians and other experts deem appropriate. Data provided in the investigational new drug (IND) application allow FDA staff to determine whether it is probably safe to market the investigational drug to humans and whether the anticipated specified therapeutic action is likely to outweigh anticipated adverse reactions. To market the drug effectively, the selected measures should address additional outcomes that demonstrate the investigational drug's value to clinicians and patients in practice.[1-5]

This chapter provides an overview of the measurement process used in a clinical drug trial. It focuses on the choice of measures used to assess the value of the investigational drug (Question 14) and the system used to measure, collect, and interpret the data (Question 15).

The basic approach to measuring and interpreting the important effects of an investigational drug is outlined in Figure 5-1. While standard approaches exist, the investigators may develop their own measurement approaches or modify existing ones. The process usually begins with a choice of study objectives. Based on these objectives, a set of measures is selected. Multiple objectives frequently require a greater number of measures. Investigators usually select the measures from a set previously developed in earlier research on the disease being studied or, if no suitable measures are available, develop their own. The measures are chosen primarily because of their coverage of the concept being measured (i.e., validity) and their repeatability (i.e., reliability). Typically, measures are chosen to assess the clinical efficacy of the drug and its relative safety. Recently, however, the measurement of outcomes has been expanded to examine humanistic outcomes such as quality of life and economic outcomes such as cost–benefit impact.[1,6–13]

**Figure 5-1** An Overview of the Measurement Process

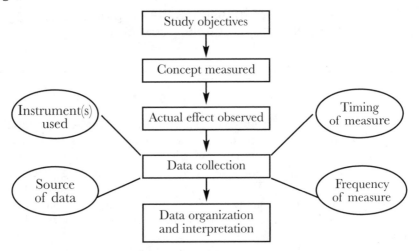

Once the measures are developed or selected, the investigators establish the system to collect and interpret the data. The measurement system usually involves establishing a plan that outlines

- when the effect is to be measured,

- how often and where the data will be acquired, and

- what measuring instrument(s) will be used.

This plan is usually part of a clinical development protocol for the investigational drug and is reviewed and monitored by the FDA throughout the drug approval process. Nevertheless, the process is still prone to biases if not properly organized and implemented (*see* Chapter 6, Questions 16 and 17).

Even if protocol deviations are minimized, the trial results could be interpreted in a biased manner by the study investigators (*see* Chapter 8, Questions 20 and 21).

## ☑ 14. Are the drug outcome measures clearly described and suitable?

Reports describing clinical drug trials should clearly and comprehensively explain the measures used to evaluate the drug treatment effects. The typical approach to measuring the expected outcomes is shown in Figure 5-2.[6,14–17]

**Figure 5-2** General Approach to Assessing the Investigational Drug's Outcomes

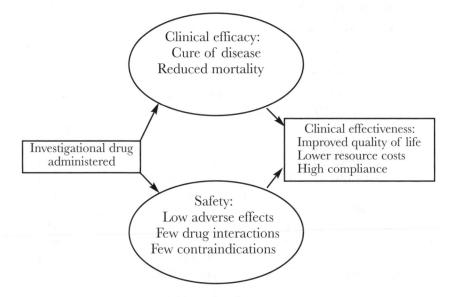

As indicated in Figure 5-2, the measurement process begins after the administration of the test drug. The primary focus is to evaluate the drug's efficacy by assessing whether it cures the disease being studied and reduces mortality. The other important focus is to establish the investigational drug's safety by monitoring adverse drug events (ADEs) and possible contraindications. While both measures are important in clinical drug trials, measurements of clinical efficacy tend be more numerous in later clinical trials (phases III and IV). The reason is that the investigational drugs tested at that point are considered relatively safe after undergoing a rigorous safety screening in the previous phase I and II clinical trials. Thus, many new ADEs are not expected. In addition, the type of ADE occurring with an investigational drug is unpredictable (especially after its basic safety profile is established) and is difficult to measure.[1,18,19]

After efficacy and safety have been established, the investigational drug's effectiveness can be measured. Drug effectiveness is the utility of the drug in practice. Clinical drug trials in the premarketing phase focus on demonstrating the investigational drug's efficacy, whereas drug effectiveness becomes a primary focus of postmarketing studies. The evaluation of drug effectiveness may involve three additional sets of measures: quality of life, proper resource utilization, and medication compliance.[1,2,4,20]

In addition to choosing which outcomes to measure, investigators should determine the appropriate endpoint of the outcome. The most important clinical endpoints are either cure of the disease or reduced mortality. However, the use of these measures, especially in most studies of chronic nonlife-threatening conditions, is difficult due to

- ethical considerations,

- the expected length of time for outcome to occur,

- the large sample sizes needed to capture the relatively uncommon event (especially mortality), and

- the resources required to ensure that the outcome could be attributed to the investigational drug.

Thus, most investigators choose to use intermediate clinical outcomes or surrogate endpoints. Intermediate clinical outcomes such as the relief of symptoms attributed to the disease state or an ADE, prevention of disease progression, or improved physical movement, are usually indirectly related to cure of the disease. Surrogate endpoints are biological or biochemical markers thought to represent disease progression that can be detected through laboratory tests. Examples are the biochemical marker cardiac Treponin T used in the treatment of myocardial infarction and plasma HIV-1 RNA used to assess AIDS therapy.[1,21–26]

Another issue is selecting the number of outcomes measured, especially in the assessment of drug efficacy. The high cost of clinical drug research dictates use of multiple clinical outcomes. One outcome is usually designated as the primary focus while the others are considered secondary. This approach does increase the probability of identifying false differences between the investigational drug and the control. The problem is more serious if no differences are observed between the experimental and control treatment on the primary outcome measure but are noted on a secondary one.[12,13,27]

A typical measurement approach (Table 5-1) was used during a clinical drug trial that compared the effectiveness of amoxicillin with that of cefaclor in urinary tract infections. As indicated in Table 5-1, the measures of clinical efficacy appear to be emphasized more than the measures of safety or effectiveness. There are three measures of drug efficacy compared to two for drug safety and one for drug effectiveness. In addition, the primary outcome measure is the use of urine cultures to assess eradication of bacteria. This widely accepted standard was performed more often than any other measure. Laboratory tests are an acceptable measure of ADEs but they were done only twice and are only indirect measures of drug toxicity. Patient interviews for the reporting of possible toxic symptoms were performed only at the end of the trial. Two measures were used for medication compliance but were performed only at the end. [17,28–32]

**Table 5-1** Measures Used to Assess Drug Outcomes in the Treatment of Urinary Tract Infections[28]

| Concept | Effect Measured | Frequency of Measurement |
|---|---|---|
| Clinical efficacy | Bacteria in urine | Performed at four different time intervals |
| | Relief of symptoms | Patient self-report at the end of treatment |
| | Antibiotic susceptibility | Cultured bacteria isolates at the beginning of trial |
| Drug safety | Laboratory abnormalities | Before and after the trial |
| | Patient report of symptoms | At the end of the trial |
| Drug effectiveness (medication compliance) | Remaining drug quantity | At the end of the trial |

## Clinical Efficacy

Once the general safety of the investigational drug is established in phase I and II research, the primary focus is then to assess the drug's clinical efficacy.[1,20,22,24,25,33–35] Although sometimes used interchangeably with the term drug effectiveness, drug efficacy represents a different research objective.

**Drug efficacy:** the extent to which the investigational drug produces a beneficial result under ideal conditions.

**Drug effectiveness:** the extent to which the investigational drug produces a clinical benefit under the usual practice situation.

Drug efficacy is usually established with double-blind placebo-controlled trials, whereas drug effectiveness studies involve different research features such as active controls, open-label studies, or case-control designs. Clinical efficacy should be established first before issues of effectiveness are examined.[1]

Measuring clinical efficacy involves focusing on the primary outcomes, which would be reduced mortality or cure. These outcomes are not generally studied in most trials because of ethical or practical concerns. Thus, most investigators select intermediate clinical outcomes or surrogate measures to assess drug efficacy[20,22,24,25,35] (Table 5-2).

**Table 5-2** Examples of Indirect Measures Used to Assess Drug Efficacy

| Desired Observed Effect | Type of Outcome | Examples |
| --- | --- | --- |
| Improvement in disease signs | Intermediate clinical outcome | Reduction in diastolic blood pressure |
| Prevention of structural damage | Intermediate clinical outcome | Radiological evidence of reduced inflammation in rheumatoid arthritis |
| Reduction in disease symptoms | Intermediate clinical outcome | Relief of headache pain |
| Remission of disease | Intermediate clinical outcome | Temporary elimination of inflammation of spinal cord in multiple sclerosis |
| Alteration of biological marker | Surrogate endpoint | Increase in $CD_4$ cell counts for AIDS patients |

While indirect outcome measures are easier to use and less expensive, they can produce misleading results. Drug efficacy could be overemphasized. Thus, it is not unusual for a test drug that showed promising therapeutic benefits in premarketing clinical research utilizing these indirect measures to be viewed as less useful when other, more direct measures are used in practice.[1]

Assessing the efficacy of an investigational drug involves multiple measures or one primary measure. There are no standard approaches, and the choice varies with the type of disease. Multiple measures usually provide a more thorough coverage of the outcome, which may improve the validity of the findings. These measures may be viewed separately or as part of a composite. However, there are limitations.[21,22,34]

An example is the evaluation of the therapeutic effect of drug treatment for irritable bowel syndrome (IBS). Because IBS is associated with many GI symptoms, investigators often measure drug effectiveness by using an extensive battery of specific tests (15 or more) of poor individual quality or an overall measure that combines numerous single measures. Neither of these approaches is desirable. The ideal set of measures would assess improvement in the important clinical features of the disease (e.g., relief of abdominal cramping or less frequent watery bowel movements) and in patient attitudes or feelings. The best evidence would be significant improvement in measures of patient feelings and most efficacy measures, especially if the pattern made clinical sense. If significant improvements were found in only a few specific measures, then conclusions regarding the drug's effectiveness would be tentative at best.[34]

## Safety

The importance of documenting the safety[18,19,23,29,30,36–42] of the investigational drug product is equal to that of drug efficacy. The measurement of drug safety is a broad approach that includes measuring all aspects of the drug's effects and all efforts to collect toxicity information. Measuring safety is difficult because of a lack of understanding regarding why ADEs occur. Unlike the few and generally well-defined outcome measures for therapeutic effects, there could be many possible ADEs that need to be monitored. In addition, the assessment of ADEs is often viewed as of secondary importance to the investigators and less attention is devoted to effectively measuring ADEs when developing the trial design.[18,19,29,39,41]

A first step toward safety monitoring is determining what to measure. Drug safety can be divided into two types of ADEs: those that occur commonly and are expected and those that are occur infrequently and are unpredictable. Common nonspecific ADEs such as nausea, vomiting, and dizziness are usually monitored in all clinical drug trials. Others specific to the test drug are usually based on its expected pharmacological effects and are dose related. Examples of these types of reactions are liver or kidney damage, GI bleeding, or inflammation of the heart muscle. Both nonspecific and specific common ADEs occur because the dose exceeds a study patient's tolerance or there is unusual individual susceptibility to the drug due to genetic factors (e.g., slower metabolism), concurrent diseases, or concomitant medications.[18,19,29,39,41]

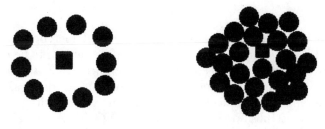

*Common ADEs are easier to identify than infrequent ones.*

The common ADEs are expected and comprise the typical safety profile of the investigational drug once it completes all phases of premarketing clinical research. The less frequent and unexpected ADEs are difficult to detect through the usual trial design. These unpredictable, idiosyncratic events appear unrelated to drug dosage or pharmacological activity. Although relatively rare, these events comprise many of the more serious ADEs. They do not usually improve with dose reduction and are more difficult to separate from the underlying disease. Because these events are rare and atypical, it is difficult to recognize and avoid them (or to establish a system to measure them). In fact, the ability of a drug to cause a relatively rare ADE may only be observed after the drug has been available for several years and used by many patients. Although their mechanism is not clear, it is probable that these ADEs are more likely to occur in genetically susceptible subgroups of patients. Examples of such reactions are drug allergies, anaphylaxis, or blood disorders.[18,19,29,39,41]

Developing a system to measure safety in a clinical drug trial is a challenge. ADEs are difficult to recognize if they are nonspecific or unexpected and may be confused with concurrent illnesses or other general symptoms. Consequently, many ADEs go undetected. To offset this problem, criteria have been established[37] to standardize the approach to detecting these reactions. The criteria include determining

- onset of the ADE compared to administration of the drug,

- course of the ADE after discontinuation of the drug,

- course of the ADE without discontinuation of the drug,

- patient response when the drug is readministered,

- presence of clinical signs and symptoms characteristic of the ADE,

- presence of patient risk factors that could precipitate the ADE,

- presence of concurrent drugs that could precipitate the ADE,

- possible nondrug factors that could precipitate the ADE, and

- specific tests for the ADE used.

In addition to establishing a standard method to detect ADEs, efforts have been made to define the specific reactions to be detected. One approach is the use of "consensus conferences." Consensus conferences involve participants responsible for evaluating drug safety such as regulatory officials, healthcare practitioners, and drug manufacturers meeting to establish precise criteria for identifying ADEs. Examples of the types of definitions developed by a consensus conference for drug-induced reduction of white blood cells (agranulocytosis)[37] are as follows:

- White blood cell (WBC) count was normal before the drug was administered.

- WBC count returns to normal after the drug was discontinued.

- Other blood factors (e.g., red blood cells, platelets) are normal during drug administration.

Regardless of the system used to detect ADEs, the length of the clinical drug trial has to be sufficient to assess both their expected and unexpected occurrence. ADEs occur relatively infrequently and are more likely to be identified as the length of the clinical drug trial increases. The duration of observation is particularly important for drugs administered for extended periods, such as investigational drugs developed to treat hypertension or congestive heart failure. Long-term trials are usually performed after the drug is approved for marketing and are better sources for rare, unexpected, or unpredictable ADEs.[18,19,23,29,30,36,38–42]

Once ADEs attributed to the test drug are detected, the investigator needs to develop an appropriate approach to comparing the results with the control treatment. Although rigorous statistical methods are required by the FDA to examine these differences, the comparison is difficult and can result in a safety analysis that is technically sound but of limited value to healthcare practitioners.[18,19,23,29,30,36,38–42]

Currently, the most commonly used method for comparing the safety profiles of two treatments is to compare the incidence rates of each individual ADE. If the sample sizes are adequate, the ADE's severity is compared as well. An example is the comparison of the incidence of nausea that occurred with the investigational drug and the control treatment. Such a comparison possesses all the desirable statistical properties assuming that a sufficient number of events occurred in each category. Unfortunately, comparison problems occur when the number of individual ADEs is so small that statistical analysis would be inappropriate. In these cases, the investigator should present the distribution of effects without a statistical comparison or should develop a composite score. Neither approach effectively compares the safety profile of the investigational drug to the control treatment.[18,19,23,29,30,36,38–42]

In fact, the use of composite scores could be misleading. While combining individual rates into a composite score enhances the statistical comparison, this approach may be unsuitable because the actual ADEs are too different. For example, combining ADEs such as dizziness, nausea, elevated liver enzymes, and radiological evidence of inflammation into a composite measure may be inappropriate.[18]

## Clinical Effectiveness

As indicated in Figure 5-2, demonstrating the investigational drug's clinical effectiveness [1,4,5,29,33,43,44] should be the ultimate goal of a clinical drug trial. Effectiveness is based on drug efficacy and is the extent to which the investigational drug, under conditions common in practice, produces a clinical benefit acceptable to individuals or organizations (e.g., patients, healthcare practitioners, healthcare organizations). Thus, research focuses on measuring the investigational drug's effect on quality of life, resource utilization, and medication compliance rather than on clinical efficacy and safety. Nevertheless, the investigational drug's clinical efficacy and safety must be established before effectiveness can be demonstrated.

Regulatory requirements have resulted in a relatively standardized approach to establishing drug efficacy and safety. A similar standard does not exist for drug effectiveness. Research designs vary significantly and involve both randomized and nonrandomized control trials, blind and unblind conditions, and small sets of similar patients or large groups of diverse patient populations. The lack of a consistent standard makes the evaluation of drug effectiveness more difficult than evaluating drug efficacy and safety.

### Quality of life

Health-related quality of life (HRQOL), an increasingly used outcome measure, is often referred to as a "humanistic" measure because it addresses human values instead of clinical outcomes. HRQOL measures patients' response beyond the typical measures of clinical efficacy and safety.[1,2,45–49] This expanded experience in assessing the value of the investigational drug has become increasingly important because of

- the aging population and the increasing prevalence of chronic diseases;

- the need to evaluate healthcare technologies with respect to individual and societal values; and

- the recognition of the value of patient perceptions in measuring drug effects.

The conceptual definition of HRQOL for a clinical drug trial refers to patients' appraisals of their current level of functioning and satisfaction with their health status. The concept, therefore, can be considered synonymous with patients' subjective assessment of the effectiveness of the investigational drug on their health. This personal perception is considered beyond the self-report of the presence and severity of symptoms associated with the disease or the test drug. Rather, it represents patients' descriptive views of their reaction to the drug therapy and the relative changes in their health status.[1,2,45–49]

The assessment of HRQOL is usually done with generic or specific health profile questionnaires. They measure health-related quality of life and well-being across multiple health domains or in areas that the patient has identified as important. Examples of domains are emotional well-being, social distress, and physical impairments. Generally each domain is assessed on a separate scale represented by an unweighted numerical value (or score).[2,47]

The choice of whether to use a generic health or specific disease instrument depends on the investigator and on instrument availability. Generic instruments are generally available and allow comparisons with patients suffering from other diseases and taking other drugs but may not focus adequately on the area of interest for a specific investigational drug. Specific instruments are likely to detect subtle changes in patient status, but they are not comprehensive, do not allow comparisons with patients suffering from other diseases, and may not be available for certain populations or drug therapy.[2,47]

Another tool for assessing HRQOL is the patient preference questionnaire. This approach focuses on quantifying the dimensions of health and providing a single numerical expression of health status referred to as a global index or utility score. Such utility scores generally range from 0.0 to 1.0 where 0.0 = death and 1.0 = perfect health. Combining utility units with the cost of an intervention results in a cost–utility score that the patient or the healthcare practitioner can use to decide on drug therapy.[2]

While health profile questionnaires measure changes in patient functional status and satisfaction attributable to the investigational drug, patient preference questionnaires focus on society and the societal allocation of healthcare resources. The quantification of the patient responses to these questionnaires allows comparison of the impact of an intervention on HRQOL to the impact of other treatments for the same condition and/or to other treatments for different conditions. Both types of questionnaires may be ineffective at detecting small but important clinical changes experienced by the patient. In addition, patient preference questionnaires vary in the approach used to measure patient preferences (e.g., standard gamble, time trade-off, or use of a rating scale).[2,47,49]

Besides the choice of instrument, the specific manner in which HRQOL is measured depends on the trial design. HRQOL measures are often used to supplement drug efficacy and safety measures and may add an unreasonable burden to patients or investigators in trials with a complicated measurement system. However, in those cases where HRQOL is the primary outcome measure, patient and staff time and other resources should be devoted to that effort. Regardless of the trial objectives, the questionnaire should be brief and simple.[2]

The phase of the trial in which HRQOL measurement is introduced is based on the judgment of the investigators. In small-scale phase II trials, HRQOL may seem unimportant. However, dramatic differences in the investigational drug's efficacy and safety may become apparent in the early research phases, and investigators may decide it is unethical to randomize patients in future trials. Therefore, pretesting the HRQOL measure on the specific population enrolled in phase II clinical trials provides insight into the investigational drug's utility in practice. In addition, evaluation of these data from the pilot study demonstrate both the feasibility of undertaking HRQOL assessment and the extent to which the study's design may require modification to accommodate it.[2]

Unlike many measures of drug safety and efficacy, the cultural perspective of the patient affects HRQOL questionnaires. Culturally adapting an HRQOL questionnaire indicates that the language and meaning within the instrument are consistent with that part of the target population represented by different ethnic groups or nationalities. The approach used most commonly is to translate a measure from one culture to another and to use focus groups for critical evaluation of the translation.[2]

Although there is no universal definition of HRQOL, the purpose of this measure is multifold. First, it provides information about how patients feel about drug therapies and may be an independent predictor of important clinical outcomes such as medication compliance, morbidity and condition severity, and mortality. Second, these data may provide valuable insights into the natural history and progression of the condition or disease. Third, it appeals to the healthcare practitioner's desire for the most effective drug therapy, and it allows the investigator to characterize the impact of a given condition or disease in terms of clinically relevant humanistic attributes likely to be understood by the subject. Finally, it may be used to distinguish between therapies that appear to be equally efficacious and equally safe and may be potentially useful at promoting the drug product by providing data on how a treatment influences an individual's daily functioning.[1,2,45–49]

### Resource use

Measuring a drug's impact on the patient's utilization of healthcare resources[44,50–52] is the focus of a type of research known as pharmacoeconomics. Pharmacoeconomics describes and analyzes the costs of drug therapy to patients, healthcare practitioners, health organizations, and society as a whole. This research identifies, measures, and compares the costs (i.e., resources consumed) and consequences of pharmaceutical products and services. Pharmacoeconomics employs various tools to examine the impact (desirable and undesirable) of alternative drug therapies and other medical interventions. The common types of tools are shown in Table 5-3.

The key feature of these analytic tools is the cost of the drug and the health services provided. Thus, the fundamental goal of researchers conducting pharmacoeconomic evaluations is to identify and compare the "opportunity costs" of the investigational drug compared to an alternative treatment. Comparing such costs is difficult in most clinical drug trials because it requires that all resources attributable to administering the investigational drug and the alternate treatment be included. Such costs include not only the relatively easy-to-identify expenses associated with administering the drug product and alternative treatment (e.g., cost of supplies and medical services) but also the more difficult assessment of the time needed by patients, caregivers, and healthcare practitioners to administer and monitor therapy.[44,50–52]

Researchers should identify all relevant outcome and resource costs of the test drug and the control treatment to develop an adequate comparison of resource utilization. The outcomes may be intermediate or final endpoints and may include both the benefits (clinical efficacy) and costs (ADEs) associated with receiving the investigational drug or the

**Table 5-3** Common Analytic Tools in Pharmacoeconomic Research[50,51]

| Analytic Tool | Description | Examples |
|---|---|---|
| Cost–benefit | Costs and consequences of drug therapy measured in dollars and results expressed as a net benefit-to-cost ratio | Comparing the costs of intravenous administration of the investigational drug (e.g., patient/health professional time, cost of supplies) with the costs associated with not using the drug (e.g., increased hospital days, more physician visits) |
| Cost–effectiveness | Costs needed to achieve a particular outcome compared with the success at reaching the outcome | Comparison of the costs required for an antibiotic to cure a urinary tract infection |
| Cost–utility | Consequences of drug therapy (e.g., quality of life) measured in terms of patient preference or the quality of the result | Patient preferences for the costs associated with receiving a chemo-therapeutic agent (e.g., nausea, increased infections) vs. not taking the drug (e.g., decreased years of life) |
| Cost–minimization | Costs of therapeutically equal drugs compared with the intent of selecting the less costly drug | Selection of an HMG-COA inhibitor (assumed to be therapeutically similar) on the basis of product costs |

control treatment. However, the challenge is to establish a suitable measure of resource use based on estimated costs. These costs can be divided into direct and indirect expenses. Direct costs are usually considered those related to administering and monitoring the effects of the investigational drug, such as expenses associated with drug products and supplies, physician visits, diagnostic tests, and hospitalizations. Other related costs that often are not estimated include such items as the expense of childcare and transportation to the trial site. Indirect costs are often more difficult to quantify and represent the value of the changes in patient health status and productivity. Both direct and indirect costs must be applicable to most clinical practice settings and based on reliable data sources.[44,50–52]

Unlike the standardized measures for assessing drug efficacy and safety, there is no consensus on the best way to estimate the cost of the resources used. A review of 181 articles about clinical trials that included a cost analysis (which included other interventions in addition to drug therapy) revealed a significant variation on how investigators estimated costs. Only about 70% of the articles reported estimates for the total treatment cost. Cost of labor was included in 42% of the articles and cost of supplies in 32%. The authors of the review concluded that published estimates of the costs of clinical interventions varied significantly depending on the methods used. Most estimates appeared to be too low, ignoring important items such as start-up and general overhead costs.[53]

The ideal time to perform an economic analysis of the resource costs would be in phase III clinical trials.[44,51,52] This approach would provide important economic data to promote the investigational drug's value to patients, healthcare practitioners, and medical care organizations. However, there are significant challenges to measuring the costs of the investigational drug in a clinical drug trial. They include

- limited generalizability,

- difficulty in evaluating costs of infrequently occurring incidents such as rare ADEs, and

- cost estimations of intermediate endpoints instead of final health outcomes.

In addition to the challenges of using the cost information collected from the clinical drug trial, there are logistical matters that complicate research, possibly increasing the cost and time of the trial and the perceived burden on investigators and patients. The economic analysis may hinder patient recruitment due to confidentiality issues, and data collection may become more complex and time consuming.[44,51,52]

Like measures of HRQOL, cost analysis of the resources devoted to the administration of the investigational drug in the clinical practice setting is important in determining the effectiveness of the drug. It presents an additional perspective on the drug utility by examining the costs to administer and monitor it. In addition, it provides additional information to compare different treatments.

### Compliance

Although sometimes considered a protocol deviation (*see* Chapter 6, Question 16), measuring patient compliance[32,54–58] is also appropriate for investigational drugs administered to ambulatory patients and for those drugs used for chronic diseases. It is an important measure of drug effectiveness because taking a drug properly is a necessary condition for most other outcomes measured. In addition, it is an efficient use of a valuable resource (i.e., the drug product). Many compliance measures are limited in their ability to estimate compliance or are difficult to implement in clinical drug trials. The advantages and disadvantages of some measures of medication compliance are shown in Table 5-4.

**Table 5-4** Various Measures of Medication Compliance [32,56–58]

| Measure | Advantages | Disadvantages |
|---|---|---|
| Clinical outcomes | Good measure of the ultimate goal of medication compliance | May not accurately estimate behavior due to poor correlation between clinical outcomes and drug administration |
| Physician estimate | Easy to use | Overestimates compliance due to poor communication with patient |
| Pill counts (visual or electronic observation) | Gives an estimate of the minimum amount of drug taken by patients | Does not determine exactly how the patient took the medication and tends to overestimate compliance |
| Prescription refill records | Gives an estimate of the minimum amount of drug taken by patient | Does not determine exactly how the patient took the medication and tends to overestimate compliance due to poor record keeping |
| Self-report | Easy to use general estimate of admitted noncompliers | Overestimates compliance due to patient response bias and poor recall |
| Serum drug levels | Good measure of presence of drug in body | May not accurately estimate compliance behavior due to poor correlation between drug administration and serum levels |

Identifying the extent of noncompliance provides valuable insight into the patient's attitudes toward the drug and medication-taking behavior. In addition, the likelihood of better compliance may be an important consideration when the investigational drug is compared with other possible treatments. In addition, assessing compliance behavior is another way of monitoring the efficient use of the investigational drug.

## ☑ 15. Is the system of measuring the drug outcomes appropriate and adequately described?

As indicated in Figure 5-1, the study objectives determine what outcomes are measured and the actual effects to be observed. Once these measures have been established, investigators need to develop an effective system for collecting and interpreting relevant data. This system involves

■ selecting reliable, valid, and sensitive measures;

- developing a comprehensive system of data collection; and

- forming an unbiased approach to organizing and interpreting the information collected.

## Reliability and Validity

Most measures are approximations of the drug's effect because the specific outcomes often cannot be measured directly. The indirect approach makes the measurement process prone to two types of errors: those that occur in an unpredictable manner (i.e., random error) and those that occur in a biased, predictable fashion (i.e., systematic error). An example of a random error would be the subjective evaluation of lung X-rays to assess the effectiveness of antitubercular drugs. The evaluation may be unpredictable because of a lack of consensus about what type of radiological evidence represents a "cure" for tuberculosis.[6,14,59]

In contrast, systematic errors are illustrated by the use of observers who anticipate a patient's response to drug treatment. Investigators with preconceived notions about a drug's effectiveness are more likely to be influenced by those impressions when interpreting the results. Both types of measurement errors influence the evaluation of efficacy and safety, but systematic errors are usually more damaging.[6,14,59]

Both random and systematic measurement errors are reduced by ensuring that the most reliable and valid measures are used. A measurement's reliability is defined as producing the same result when used multiple times, assuming that the patient's status has not changed. The evaluation of the reliability or reproducibility of a measure should focus on the agreement among a set of repeated measures on the same patient. Assuming that no change occurs in health or physical status, the measurement should yield basically the same result when used at different times. An example of a reliable measure would be two measures of a patient's blood pressure taken a month apart producing similar readings if the patient's hypertension has not changed. Because some degree of variation is anticipated, reliable measures are not expected to provide identical results each time.[6-8]

Another term that is closely related to reliability is precision. In statistical terms, precision refers to the grouping of the measurements around a certain mean point. Closely grouped data are considered more precise than data points spread widely apart.[60,61]

A measurement's validity is defined as the extent to which a measure assesses what it is supposed to measure. The assessment of a measure's validity is more difficult than assessing its reliability because there is usually no absolute standard against which the measure's performance can be compared. Thus, determination of validity is more complicated and depends on a clear idea of what is supposed to be measured. For example, typical measures of clinical efficacy for the antibiotic treatment of urinary tract infections would be the in vitro effect on susceptible organisms, absence of harmful bacteria in the urine, or relief of associated symptoms. From a clinical standpoint, the most valid measure would be the relief of the symptoms because that is the standard most acceptable to patients and healthcare practitioners.[9–11,62]

Accuracy is a term used in statistical analysis similar to validity. A measure is more accurate when it closely approximates the true value than when its approximations are far apart. A test or measure that is not reliable cannot be valid. However, invalid measures can be reliable.[60,61]

Common approaches used to enhance the reliability and validity of the measurements and reduce the likelihood of error are the use of double-blind techniques, frequent measurement times, and multiple measures. Their use to measure a drug's efficacy and safety should be explained comprehensively and clearly in any description of the trial. A double-blind design minimizes the effect of two major sources of systematic measurement error: the bias of the investigator in interpreting events and the bias of the patient in reporting results. If the type of drug treatment under investigation prevents blinding of the investigator, observers independent from the research team should be used to measure trial outcomes. [59,62,63]

Measurement reliability is established using frequent measurement times, assuming that the measure shows consistent results each time. One way to demonstrate reliability statistically is through the assessment of test–retest reliability, determined by using the measure at multiple points in the clinical drug trial and examining the statistical association. Multiple measures of the same outcome can also be used to establish reliability if the single measures are combined into a composite score and its internal consistency examined. Both approaches to reliability assessment are examined numerically by a scale ranging from 0.0 to 1.0, with 1.0 considered a perfect match.[2]

Measurement validity could be enhanced by multiple measures of the same outcome, which represents the concept of convergent validity. The validity is based on the assessment of the degree to which each measure is associated with each other and not associated to measures of different outcomes. Multiple measures are used to assess all-important aspects of the patient's response and to avoid missing any evidence of benefit.[2,10,64]

The use of multiple measures of the same outcome is illustrated in a trial that examined the effectiveness of intravenous infusion of gamma globulin (immune globulin) in the treatment of acute Kawasaki syndrome. Symptoms such as fever, rash, swollen and red hands and feet, conjunctivitis, and inflammation of the mucous membranes characterize this syndrome. Multiple measures were used to assess clinical efficacy: presence or absence of coronary abnormalities, temperature, laboratory indexes of systemic inflammation, and serum IgG levels.[65]

Unfortunately, the use of multiple measures can be detrimental if the strategy relies more on the number of measures used than on the quality of each measure. Use of a large number of poor measures may result in different findings, which could make assessment of the drug effect difficult. The choice of which measures to believe can be confusing, especially if they differ in quality. A better solution would be to carefully choose measures that are most relevant, sensitive to change, and not duplicative of other measures used.[10]

## Sensitivity

The measure's sensitivity for assessing a trial outcome refers to its responsiveness to detect clinically significant changes over time. Clinical drug trials often fail to show a particular result because the measurements used are not sufficiently sensitive to detect changes. In the treatment of arthritis, trials that use radiographic findings to assess joint healing often fail to reveal success compared with more sensitive measures such as counting the number of improved joints. Lack of sensitivity is a particular problem with measures of health-related quality of life.[2,64]

The sensitivity or responsiveness of a measure can be enhanced through the careful choice of measures and multiple testing times. In addition, the results can be compared with similar changes in other measures of the same concept to determine if detected changes (or lack of detection) are associated. However, extremely sensitive measures may also cause problems. Such measures are likely to detect small differences between the experimental and control groups that could be clinically unimportant. The overly optimistic investigator may choose to interpret and report these differences as clinically important when, in fact, they are not.[2,66]

Determining the measure's sensitivity for detecting changes should not be confused with its sensitivity as a screening tool. Measures as screening tools are used in the patient enrollment process to screen patients for certain factors: presence of a specific symptom, surrogate marker, or set of behaviors. The sensitivity of the measure for this function reflects its ability to detect the factor in patients who truly have it. A highly sensitive measure for this application would detect every patient who has the factor in a pool of patients that includes those without the factor.[2,67,68]

A related concept is the specificity of the measure. Specificity refers to the ability of the measure to identify patients who do not have the factor. Thus, measures with high sensitivity and high specificity would identify only the patients who have the factor and exclude patients who do not.[2,67,68]

## Data Collection

Data collection procedures[3,19,69,70] must be designed to manage the enormous amount of data collected during the trial. It is estimated that if a study enrolls only 25 patients who visit a study site only four times, each patient visit may generate 60–100 variables, resulting in a total database of 6000–10,000 pieces of data. These data need to be collected to ensure completeness, reliability, and validity. Thus, careful planning and adherence to procedures are needed to ensure that the data are collected properly. Included in the plan should be a description of how the data will be handled statistically.

Most data collection procedures undergo a rigorous review by the various organizations involved in clinical research, such as the drug sponsor and the FDA. The data collection plan and procedures should be described thoroughly, especially the source(s) of the data, the instruments used, the timing of the measures, and how frequently they will be used. How the investigators recorded and scored the data values should be described as well. In addition, there should be a procedure for reporting serious, life-threatening, or fatal ADEs. The information provided on the ADE should be complete enough to enable the sponsor to provide the FDA with the necessary legal material.[3,19,69,70]

### Instrument(s) used and sources of data

Investigators should clearly describe the instrument(s)[2,10,59] used to measure the drug outcomes, including known reliability, validity, and sensitivity. These instruments should be consistent with those used in previous clinical research about the drug or the disease. When an instrument is used in a new population or disease from that in which it was originally developed, the modification to the different research environment should be discussed. The justification for the selection of that particular instrument should be given and supported by references, particularly if it is a relatively new tool.

The procedures regarding how the instrument is used should be standardized, especially in multicenter studies involving many investigators, to reduce bias and measurement error. Examples of instruments of measurement and procedures that should be standardized include blood pressure readings, laboratory testing, and physical examination. In most cases, qualitative (i.e., subjective) procedures such as pain sensation are much harder to standardize than are quantitative (i.e., objective) procedures such as assessing bacterial levels.

Unfortunately, clinical drug trials for the treatment of a particular medical condition often vary in the types of measures used, making comparison of the results difficult. For example, assessment of an antiarthritic drug's clinical efficacy varies depending on how the response of the inflamed joint (i.e., joint count) is measured. The drug may be more effective in a trial that measured the number of "tender" joints than in a trial that counted the number of "swollen" joints.[64] The instrument description should include

- the method used to administer the tool,

- the source of the data (self-report, face-to-face interview, laboratory tests, investigator observation),

- the time frame in which the instrument was used to measure the effect, and

- the method used to score the data.

An example of a clear description occurred in a trial comparing the effectiveness of norfloxacin with co-trimoxazole in the treatment of urinary tract infections. Therapeutic effectiveness of the two antibiotics was represented by measures of the number of bacteria eradicated in the urine (i.e., bacterial cure) and relief of symptoms associated with urinary tract infections (i.e., clinical cure). The bacterial cure was measured by a standardized urinalysis in which the urine collection scheme was specified clearly (i.e., two midstream urine specimens). The clinical cure was assessed by blind observations and physical examination. Both measures were performed four times during the trial and at the appropriate time interval for allowing the drug to reach optimal activity.[71]

### Frequency and timing of measure

The description of the data collection should provide a clear overview of the frequency and timing of each measure.[72] Screening visits, baseline laboratory evaluations, when the first day of dosing began, washout periods, and postdosing evaluations should all be discussed. Even more helpful would be a table or flowchart wherein the various measurement times can be viewed in relationship to each other. For crossover studies, the drug-free and washout periods should be defined clearly. The predrug period, which is the patient preparation phase of the clinical drug trial, should also be thoroughly described. This description includes any washout periods or placebo response evaluations used before the administration of the investigational drug or control treatment to eliminate the effects of prior drugs. In addition to the frequency and timing of the measure, the length of the measurement period should be described, including the maximum allowable time required to complete the evaluation of all patients.

### Data organization and interpretation

Data organization involves the manipulation of various forms of data into an easy to interpret format. This approach usually involves reducing objective and subjective data into various classifications that broadly represent clinical improvement, no change, or a negative effect. Although classification scales for data exist (*see* Chapter 7, Question 17), there is often no standard way to designate positive change from negative or no change. Usually, the designation is based on the consensus of the investigators or the opinion of the healthcare practitioner who uses the drug in practice. It is often difficult for study results to be accepted in areas where no consensus exists (e.g., arthritis).[72,73]

The problem of interpreting the data is worse for subjective than for objective data.[72,73] While objective data are already numerically quantified, subjective data are converted to a numerical scale for statistical analysis. This conversion is often dependent on the investigator and can be prone to bias. An example would be the numerical conversion of symptoms associated with clinical improvement. Proper standardization of the conversions is essential. For example, a scale could be created in the measure in which a numeric value is placed next to a corresponding level of the symptom. A five-point measurement scale for pain relief may have the following rating values:

1 = no pain,

2 = mild pain, about once per week,

3 = moderate pain, occurs every day

4 = moderately severe pain, feels pain daily and gets medication relief

5 = severe pain, feels pain all the time and gets no pain relief.

Regardless of the system used, there should be an explanation and justification of the method by which the clinician's words, such as "lethargy," "severe pain," or "stupor," are transformed into numbers that can be manipulated in statistical calculations.[72]

# References

1. Lasagna L. Balancing risks versus benefits in drug therapy decisions. *Clin Ther.* 1998; 20:C72–C79.

2. Berzon RA. Understanding and using health-related quality of life instruments within clinical research studies. In: Staquet MJ, Hays RD, Fayers PM, eds. *Quality of Life Assessment in Clinical Trials.* New York: Oxford University Press; 1998:3–15.

3. Kassalow LM. Statistical and data management: collaboration in clinical research. In: Gaurino RA, ed. *New Drug Approval Process: The Global Challenge.* 3rd ed. New York: Marcel Dekker; 2000:289–310.

4. Pathek DS, Escovitz A. Assuring the safe use of medications: the drug approval process and improving treatment decisions. *Clin Ther.* 1998; 20:C1–C4.

5. Decoster G, Buyse M. Clinical research after drug approval: what is needed and what is not. *Drug Info J.* 1999; 33:627–34.

6. McAuley WJ. *Applied Research in Gerontology.* New York: Van Nostrand-Reinhold, 1987:77–103.

7. Isaacs S, Michael WB. *Handbook in Research and Evaluation.* San Diego: Edits Publishers, 1976:125.

8. Speedie SM. Reliability: the accuracy of a test. *Am J Pharm Ed.* 1985; 49:76–9.

9. Kimberlin CL. Characteristics desired in tests: validity. *Am J Pharm Ed.* 1985; 49:73–85.

10. Haynes RB. How to read clinical journals. II. To learn about a diagnostic test. *CMA J.* 1981; 124:703–10.

11. Verbrugge LM. Scientific and professional allies in validity studies. In: Fowler FJ, ed. *Health Survey Research Methods*. Conference Proceedings Series. DHHS Publ. No. (PHS) 89:3447.

12. Davis CE. Secondary endpoints can be validly analyzed, even if the primary endpoint does not provide clear statistical significance. *Controlled Clin Trials*. 1997; 18:557–60.

13. Pocock SJ. Clinical trials with multiple outcomes: a statistical perspective on their design, analysis, and interpretation. *Controlled Clin Trials*. 1997; 18:530–45.

14. Cuddy PG, Elenbaas RM, Elenbaas JK. Evaluating the medical literature. Part I: abstract, introduction, methods. *Ann Emerg Med*. 1983; 12:549–55.

15. Pocock SJ. *Clinical Trials: A Practical Approach*. New York: Wiley, 1983:188–91.

16. Weintraub M. How to critically assess clinical drug trials. *Drug Ther*. 1982; (July):131–48.

17. Tugwell PX. How to read clinical journals. III. To learn the clinical course and prognosis of disease. *CMA J*. 1981; 124:869–72.

18. Chuang-Stein C, Mohberg NR. A unified approach to the analysis of safety data in clinical trials. In: Solgliero-Gilbert G, ed. *Drug Safety Assessment in Clinical Trials*. 3rd ed. New York: Marcel Dekker; 1993:235–65.

19. Peace KE. Design and analysis considerations for safety data, particularly adverse events. In: Solgliero-Gilbert G, ed. *Drug Safety Assessment in Clinical Trials*. 3rd ed. New York: Marcel Dekker; 1993:305–16.

20. Hartzema AG, Porta MS, Tilson HH. *Pharmacoepidemiology: An Introduction*. 2nd ed. Cincinnati: Harvey Whitney Books; 1991.

21. Solgliero-Gilbert G, Zubkoff-Schulz L, Ting N. The genie score: a multivariate assessment of laboratory abnormalities. In: Solgliero-Gilbert G, ed. *Drug Safety Assessment in Clinical Trials*. 3rd ed. New York: Marcel Dekker; 1993: 125–70.

22. Cannon C. Clinical perspective on the use of composite endpoints. *Controlled Clin Trials*. 1997; 18:517–29.

23. Petri H, Leufkens H, Naus J, et al. Rapid method for estimating the risk of acutely controversial side effects of prescription drugs. *J Clin Epidemiol*. 1990; 43:433–9.

24. Hammer S. Use of surrogate versus clinical markers in trials for HIV infection. *Drug Info J*. 1999; 33:347–52.

25. Liu T, Wang Q, Baxter MS, et al. Development of a statistical model for prediction of acute myocardial infarction by biochemical markers. *Drug Info J*. 1999; 33:141–8.

26. Bunker JP. The selection of endpoints in evaluative research. In: Gelijns A, ed. *Modern Methods of Clinical Investigation*. Washington, DC: National Academy Press; 1990:16–22.

27. O'Neill RT. Secondary endpoints cannot be validly analyzed if the primary endpoint does not demonstrate clear statistical significance. *Controlled Clin Trials*. 1997; 18:550–6.

28. Jaffe AC, O'Brien CA, Reed MD, et al. Randomized comparative evaluation of Augmentin® and cefaclor in pediatric skin and soft-tissue infections. *Curr Ther Res*. 1985; 38:160–8.

29. Dimenas E, Dahlof C, Olofsson B, et al. An instrument for quantifying subjective symptoms among untreated and treated hypertensives: development and documentation. *J Clin Res Pharmacoepidem*. 1990; 4:205–17.

30. Friedman LM, Furberg CD, DeMets DL. *Fundamentals of Clinical Trials*. 2nd ed. Littleton, MA: PSG Publishing, 1985:147–66.

31. Kramer MS, Shapiro SH. Scientific challenges in the application of randomized trials. *JAMA*. 1984; 252:2739–45.

32. Averbuch M, Weintraub M, Pollock DJ. Compliance assessment in clinical trials. *J Clin Res Pharmacoepidem*. 1990; 4:199–204.

33. Elwood MJ. *Critical Appraisal of Epidemiological Studies and Clinical Trials*. New York: Oxford University Press; 1998:94–114.

34. Klein KB. Controlled treatment trials in the irritable bowel syndrome: a critique. *Gastroenterology*. 1988; 95:232–41.

35. Neuhauser M, Steinijans V, Bretz F. The evaluation of multiple clinical endpoints, with application to asthma. *Drug Info J*. 1999; 20:471–7.

36. Brennan TA, Localio RJ, Laird NL. Reliability and validity of judgments concerning adverse events suffered by hospitalized patients. *Med Care.* 1989; 27:1148–58.

37. Benichou C, Danan G. Experts' opinion in causality assessment: results of consensus meetings. *Drug Info J.* 1991; 25:251–5.

38. Lydeck E, Blumenthal SJ, Guess HA. Twenty years of renal adverse experience reporting with Indocin®. *J Clin Res Pharmacoepidem.* 1990; 4:183–9.

39. Kirby D. Adverse drug events in clinical trials. In: Solgliero-Gilbert G, ed. *Drug Safety Assessment in Clinical Trials.* 3rd ed. New York: Marcel Dekker; 1993:25–38.

40. DeWitt JE, Sorofman BA. A model for understanding patient attribution of adverse drug reaction symptoms. *Drug Info J.* 1999; 33:907–20.

41. Hutchinson TA, Lane DA. Assessing methods for causality assessment of suspected adverse drug reactions. *J Clin Epidem.* 1989; 42:5–16.

42. Kitler ME. The changing face of clinical trials. *J Hypertension.* 1988; 6 (suppl 1):S73–S80.

43. FDA Center for Drug Evaluation and Research. *From Test Tube to Patient: Improving Health Through Human Drugs.* Rockville MD: Food and Drug Administration; 1999:33–40.

44. Sanchez LA. Applied pharmacoeconomics: evaluation and use of pharmacoeconomic data from literature. *Am J Health Syst Pharm.* 1999; 56:1630–40.

45. Committee on Clinical Practice Guidelines, Institute of Medicine, ed.; *Guidelines for Clinical Practice.* Washington DC: National Academy Press; 1992.

46. Ki FYC, Chow S-C. Statistical justification for the use of composite scores in quality of life assessment. *Drug Info J.* 1995; 29:715–28.

47. Anderson RB. What does it mean: anchoring psychosocial quality of life scale score changes with reference to concurrent changes in reported symptom distress. *Drug Info J.* 1999; 33:445–53.

48. Stewart AL, Greenfield S, Wells K, et al. Functional status and well-being of patients with chronic conditions. *JAMA.* 1989; 262:909–13.

49. Rajagoplan R, Anderson RT, Sherertz EF. Quality of life evaluation in chronic lichen sclerosis for improved medical care. *Drug Info J.* 1999; 33:577–84.

50. Bootman JL, Townsend RJ, McGhan WF. *Principles of Pharmacoeconomics.* Cincinnati: Harvey Whitney Books; 1991:3–17.

51. Motheral BR, Jackson TR. Understanding and evaluating original research articles. *J Am Pharm Assoc.* 1999; 39(6):759–74.

52. Baker AM, Goldberg RJ, Kaniecki DJ. Economic analysis in clinical trials: practical considerations. *Drug Info J.* 1999; 33:1053–60.

53. Bala AE, Kretschmer RAC, Gnann W, et al. Interpreting cost analyses of clinical interventions. *JAMA.* 1998; 279(1): 54–7.

54. Kastrissios H, Blaschke TF. Medication compliance as a feature in drug development. *Ann Rev Pharmacol Toxicol.* 1997; 37:451–75.

55. Nichol MB, Venturini F, Sung JC. A critical evaluation of methodology of the literature on medication compliance. *Ann Pharmacol.* 1999; 33:531–40.

56. Meichenbaum D, Turk DC. *Facilitating Treatment Adherence: A Practitioner's Guidebook.* New York: Plenum Press; 1987:31–40.

57. Roth HP. Measurement of compliance. *Pat Educ Coun.* 1987; 10:107–16.

58. Brooks CM, Richards JM, Martin B, et al. Assessing adherence to asthma and inhaler regimens: a psychometric analysis of adult self-report scales. *Med Care.* 1994; 32:298–307.

59. Gehlbach SH. *Interpreting the Medical Literature: A Clinician's Guide.* New York, Macmillan; 1988:83–95.

60. De Muth JE; *Basic Statistics and Pharmaceutical Statistical Applications.* New York: Marcel Dekker; 1999.

61. Bolton S; *Pharmaceutical Statistics: Practical and Clinical Applications.* New York: Marcel Dekker; 1990.

62. Polk RE, Hepler CD. Controversies in antimicrobial therapy: critical analysis of clinical trials. *Am J Hosp Pharm.* 1986; 43:630–40.

63. Franks P. Clinical trials. *Fam Med.* 1988; 20:443–8.

64. Felson DT, Anderson JJ, Meenan RF. Time for changes in design, analysis, and reporting of rheumatoid arthritis clinical trials. *Arth Rheum.* 1990; 33:140–9.

65. Newburger JW, Takahashi M, Beiser AS, et al. A single intravenous infusion of gamma globulin as compared with four infusions in the treatment of acute Kawasaki syndrome. *N Engl J Med.* 1991; 324:1633–9.

66. Horwitz RI. Complexity and contradiction in clinical trial research. *Am J Med.* 1987; 82:498–510.

67. Elwood MJ. *Critical Appraisal of Epidemiological Studies and Clinical Trials.* New York: Oxford University Press; 1998:218–44.

68. Morton RF, Hebel JR, McCarter RJ. *A Study Guide to Epidemiology and Biostatistics.* 4th ed. Gaithersburg MD: Aspen; 1996.

69. Mackintosh DR. Detection of negligence, fraud, and other bad faith efforts during field auditing of clinical trial sites. *Drug Info J.* 1996; 30:645–53.

70. Groenewoud G, Bell PJ. The need for pre-trial audits in clinical trials-an investigator's perspective. *Drug Info J.* 1995; 29:639–44.

71. Wong WT, Chan MK, Li MK, et al. Treatment of urinary tract infections in Hong Kong: a comparative study of norfloxacin and co-trimoxazole. *Scan J Inf Dis.* 1988; 56(suppl):22–7.

72. Gaurino RA. Clinical research protocols. In: Gaurino RA, ed. *New Drug Approval Process: The Global Challenge.* 3rd ed. New York: Marcel Dekker; 2000:219–46.

73. Lydick E, Yawn BP. Clinical interpretation of health-related quality of life data. In: Staquet MJ, Hays RD, Fayers PM, eds. *Quality of Life Assessment in Clinical Trials.* New York: Oxford University Press; 1998:299–314.

# Results: Protocol and Data Management Problems

**6**

---

➤☐ 16. Are all protocol deviations reported and managed appropriately?

➤☐ 17. Are all missing data and patient withdrawals analyzed properly?

---

Quite often, the first part of the results section describes the success that the investigators had in following the research plan or protocol. From a regulatory perspective, the research protocol is necessary for drug development and is vital to the drug approval process. Although essential as a regulatory requirement, a definitive research protocol is important for any clinical trial to minimize the potential for bias. Failure to follow this plan is commonly referred to as protocol deviation and includes failing to meet enrollment goals, the selection of the wrong type of patient, participants not following the research plan, the use of concurrent medications, and inappropriate awareness of the drug treatment.[1–4]

In addition to protocol deviations, investigators also need to describe their approach to data management. These concepts overlap but are subtly different. Protocol deviations represent the degree to which the investigators failed to follow the research plan and are usually reported at the beginning of the results section. Data management strategies characterize the approach used to handle patient data and are reported throughout the article. The most prominent challenge is the management of incomplete or missing data and patient withdrawals.[3,4]

This chapter provides an overview of the problems that occur when investigators are unable to follow the research plan precisely (Question 16). Also covered are problems associated with bias and how to reduce it in data collection and management (Question 17). Such problems may significantly affect results and need to be examined thoroughly by the reader when reviewing the article.

## ☑ 16. Are all protocol deviations reported and managed appropriately?

The research protocol is a comprehensive plan for the clinical drug trial that describes how the study will be performed.[1] The protocol includes specific procedures to

- protect the well-being of study subjects,
- address the medical and statistical objectives of the clinical trial,
- meet regulatory requirements, and
- adhere to sponsor policies and guidelines.

Departures from this plan are generally called protocol deviations and occur commonly, especially in relatively long-term trials or studies with complicated measures or drug administration schedules. A high incidence of protocol deviations may indicate that the trial is poorly administered, with poor cooperation from patients and investigators. A large number of protocol deviations severely compromises the data and should be avoided.[1,2,5]

Checks or audits for protocol deviations should begin early and continue throughout the study. The intent is to identify patterns and instances of data omissions, inconsistencies, and irregular relationships between measures and to determine whether the recording of the clinical observations or drug administrations is performed in a proper sequence. Protocol violations must be identified and characterized, and some explanation should be provided regarding the cause, such as the investigators' misunderstanding or misinterpretation of the protocol, indifference and sloppiness, communication problems with the patient, or, rarely, fraudulent practices.[2,5–7]

Protocol deviations are usually categorized and reported in the first part of the results section, although sometimes elsewhere, particularly if likely to bias interpretation of the results. An explanation should be given on how the impact of these deviations was minimized. Examples of the more common types of protocol deviations are shown in Table 6-1.[3,8]

### Missing Patient Enrollment Goals

Investigators often fail to enroll the optimal sample size or number of patients because of the inherent problems associated with patient enrollment. Although infrequently done, the intended sample size for the trial should be stated in the methods section along with the reasons why the goal was not achieved. This inclusion provides insight into possible biases that occurred with patient recruitment.

**Table 6-1** Examples of Protocol Deviations

| Type | Description |
| --- | --- |
| Missing patient enrollment goals | Failure to reach the projected number of subjects needed to assess the trial objectives and to generalize results |
| Selecting ineligible patients | Selecting patients who did not satisfy the selection criteria and who are likely to be unresponsive or unusually sensitive to the investigational drug |
| Failure to follow trial procedures | Unsuccessful adherence to study procedures by patients, investigators, or both |
| Unauthorized concurrent medication use | Patients taking—without the knowledge of the investigators—medication that may affect the investigational drug |
| Awareness of drug treatment | Unplanned investigator or patient awareness of the drug treatment in a blind study |

An example would be reporting that the enrollment goal was not met due to lack of patient interest. This lack of interest may reflect the patients' belief that the investigational drug would not be beneficial.[3,9-11]

A lower than expected number of patients may have a significant impact on the interpretation of the trial results because investigators rarely plan to enroll more subjects than they need. Fewer patients may result in insufficient participants in the experimental and control groups, resulting in a failure to detect true differences between the groups. In addition, the reduced number of subjects may minimize the expected heterogeneity of the trial sample and thus limit the study's generalizability (*see* Chapter 9, Question 24).

## Selecting Ineligible Patients

The presence of patients who did not meet selection criteria is often the result of poor or inappropriately administered diagnostic tests or the use of vague selection criteria. Ineffective tests are the result of poor sensitivity or selectivity (*see* Chapter 5, Question 15). Vague selection criteria make it difficult to determine who should be in the study. In either case, including ineligible subjects in the trial sometimes reflects a lack of planning, lack of understanding about the disease, or (rarely) intentional bias.[5,11]

Although clear and precise selection criteria and an effective screening test should prevent large numbers of ineligible patients from entering the trial, some patients are included by mistake. Such patients may affect the results, especially if the number of ineligible patients is relatively large. One possible effect would be the presence of a group of patients significantly different from the patients originally targeted. A less likely impact could be an alteration of the comparability of the experimental and control groups through assignment of substantially more ineligible patients to one group. The use of random assignment should reduce the likelihood of different groups. However, the potential for assigning more ineligible patients to one group increases as the sample size decreases.[3,8]

There are no clear rules regarding the handling of ineligible patients in the analysis of the reported results. Patients identified and excluded before randomization are often not listed. However, current regulatory practices require (or at least strongly suggest) that any ineligible patient assigned to a group be identified and included in the analysis. This approach is called "intention-to-treat" analysis and is also used to handle patient withdrawals.[12] Providing details about ineligible patients reveals important information regarding the efficacy and safety of the investigational drug. The details are of special importance if the patients were declared ineligible because of a prior adverse drug event (ADE) with the investigational drug or a similar compound. Reporting the number of ineligible patients also provides information about the full range of patients considered for the drug trial and may be useful when applying the trial results to patients in practice.[3,9]

## Failure to Follow Trial Procedures

The treatment and measurement procedures for clinical drug trials are very complex, and it would be surprising if 100% adherence were reported for both the patients and research team. Failure to follow every study procedure is only a problem if a systematic failure exists or many failures are reported. Examples of failures include patient noncompliance to drug therapy or nondrug treatments, inconsistent drug administration, or variable data collection efforts by the research team.

### Patient noncompliance

Patient noncompliance with medication administration guidelines is a major problem in trials involving ambulatory patients or in any trial in which patients are responsible for self-administration.[13] The failure of patients to take their medications correctly dramatically influences the interpretation of the results. Noncompliance may be due to

- a misunderstanding of the treatment instructions,

- mistakes in administration of the investigational drugs, or

- a deliberate attempt by the patient to take the medication improperly.

Noncompliance due to patient misunderstanding is usually the result of poor communication. Drug administration errors may be due to mislabeling or to dispensing the wrong medication during a clinic visit. Undesirable side effects, failed therapeutic effect, or ineffective monitoring of the patient's medication use may result in deliberate noncompliance.[3,8,14,15]

Discovering that a substantial number of patients do not comply with the trial guidelines for taking medications may indicate that the trial protocol is too difficult. In addition, reduced patient compliance in one treatment group relative to another could result in investigators making incorrect conclusions regarding observed differences. The investigators may incorrectly favor one investigational drug over another or conclude that no difference exists when one actually does.[3,8,14,15] For example, the therapeutic efficacy of an investigational drug may be overestimated because the investigator failed to account for patients who dropped out due to noncompliance. In addition, drug toxicity may be underestimated if the patients intentionally reduced the amount of medication they took. Thus, the extrapolation of trial results could be limited if the potential for noncompliance in the clinical setting is not evaluated accurately.[14,15]

In addition to reporting the number of protocol deviations due to noncompliance, investigators should also report how compliance was measured to ensure that this problem was addressed.[16] If effective measures are not feasible, one suggested approach is to measure the blood drug levels obtained in compliant patients and compare those data against blood levels for all patients.[13]

### Patient noncompliance with nondrug factors

Nondrug factors important in clinical drug trials include the type of diet and the amount of sleep required. Patient noncompliance with these factors generally does not affect the overall interpretation of the reported results, although they may be an indirect indication of noncompliance with the drug regimen or communication problems between the trial patients and the investigators.[3,8]

Compliance with nondrug factors becomes more meaningful in trials in which these factors affect the primary clinical outcome measured. An example would be the trial that investigated the efficacy of fluvastatin in hypercholesterolemia. The control group took the standard drug treatment at the time, cholestyramine. However, to control for the influences of diet on the clinical outcome (i.e., serum lipids), the patients were required to follow a rigid, standardized diet during the 18-week study.[17]

Another example is the comparison of the investigational drug with a nondrug control treatment. A clinical drug trial to demonstrate the efficacy of the blood lipid-lowering drug lovastatin illustrates this comparison. In this study, lovastatin was compared to a control group that received a regulated-fat diet for 36 weeks.[18]

### Investigator failure to administer drug

Like patient noncompliance, failure to properly administer the drug to patients by the research team may result in a biased estimation of the drug's efficacy. The likelihood of failing to administer a dose increases with the complexity and the length of the administration schedule. This problem occurred in a trial that evaluated the efficacy of sumatriptan for the treatment of migraine. In this study, sumatriptan or placebo was administered subcutaneously to patients when they were enrolled in the study and reported to the study clinic with migraine symptoms. If the headache persisted for 60 minutes after the initial administration, the patients received a second subcutaneous dose of the investigational drug or the placebo. Failure to follow the dosage schedule was reported in 24 of 639 patients (3.8%), primarily due to delayed administration of the second injection.[19]

The probability of failure to properly administer a drug increases when the administration decision is shared jointly with the patient. In one example, two cancer chemotherapy combinations, cisplatin with cyclophosphamide and cisplatin with paclitaxel, were compared in the treatment of ovarian cancer. The patients were to receive the chemotherapy every three weeks for six courses. Despite the fact that the medical staff was administering the drug, 36 of the 385 patients (9.3%) who completed the study did not receive all six courses, primarily because of drug toxicity or a lack of desire to receive the combination. In addition, the median days between treatment cycles increased in the cisplatin–cyclophosphamide group from the desired standard of 21 days after the first administration to 28 days by the sixth course of treatment.[20]

Like patient noncompliance, investigator nonadherence to the drug administration schedule can lead to a biased interpretation of the trial results because the total dose administered is less than optimal. Clinical efficacy may be underestimated. Even if clinical efficacy is established, dose-related toxicity may be underreported.

### Variations in data collection procedures or drug administration times

Data collection problems are generally due to failure of investigators to gather data at the correct time intervals or to patients missing scheduled appointments. Although such violations usually do not affect the overall interpretation of the reported results, they are important in clinical trials of certain types of drugs.[3,8] An example would be assessment of the comparative effectiveness of two inhalant bronchodilators such as albuterol and epinephrine. The duration of action of albuterol is 3–6 hours and that of epinephrine is 1–3 hours. One-hour variations in data collection could result in cases where the effects of the drugs are no longer present. Because the duration of epinephrine's effect is shorter, variations in data collection may produce results that inaccurately favor albuterol.[21]

Data collection procedures are more prone to be disregarded if the information to be collected is the joint responsibility of the investigator and the patient. An example is the measurement of health-related quality of life. This concept is usually measured through self-administered questionnaires, which are often completed away from the study site. In large-scale studies involving multiple measurement times, the likelihood of a 100% completion rate is low.[22]

## Unauthorized Concurrent Medication Use

The use of concurrent medications is common in studies with ambulatory patients, especially under conditions in which the patients are likely to suffer from other medical problems. Concurrent medications are often permitted because of the ethical need to ensure that the trial patients receive proper care for all medical conditions as well as the one being investigated. Although their use may be unrelated to the investigational drug, concurrent medications are sometimes used as part of the standard of care for the medical condition being studied to compensate for the poor efficacy of the investigational drug or to treat side effects. These drugs are often called "rescue" medications. Examples would be the use of an adjunct pain reliever such as acetaminophen in a trial assessing the safety and efficacy of an antiarthritic drug or the use of naloxone to reverse respiratory depression caused by narcotic drugs in a trial investigating the treatment of acute pain. All concurrent medications should be reported because they may mask the true effects of the investigational drug.[3,8,23]

## Awareness of Drug Treatment

Investigator or patient awareness of which drug treatment a particular patient is receiving would be a violation of protocol in double-blind clinical drug trials.[8,9,24–26] Although the problem may appear when the confidential code identifying the trial drugs is inappropriately opened or when the patient assignment scheme is improperly revealed, protocol deviations are also likely to occur when the investigational or control drugs have prominent therapeutic effects or ADEs. Investigator or patient awareness of the drug treatment procedures may significantly bias the data collection and interpretation and could represent a serious protocol deviation.

# ☑ 17. Are all missing data and patient withdrawals analyzed properly?

The amount of data collected and analyzed in a clinical drug trial is large and complex. Thus, it is not surprising that some data are lost or that the analysis may only address part of the data. The approach used to deal with missing data needs to be presented clearly to ensure that it does not significantly bias the analysis and interpretation of the results. In addition, the data presented must be consistent with the study objectives.

## Reporting Missing Data and Patient Withdrawals

All patients entered in the trial must be accounted for in the results section. The investigator should specifically state the number of patients who are missing from the analysis. The discussion should identify patients excluded during the enrollment process, that withdrew or were lost to follow-up, or that died. Also included should be the reasons why patients withdrew, such as a perceived lack of efficacy, troublesome ADEs, or non-compliance. Patients who completed the study but have missing data should also be identified and categorized. These patients include those who failed to complete the drug treatment according to protocol, received other drug treatments not specified in the protocol, or received the drug treatment at different time intervals than planned.[22]

The method(s) by which missing data are defined and analyzed must be clearly stated. Ideally, data should be discussed as well as displayed in tables and graphs. In particular, inconsistencies between the number of patients reported in figures, graphs, tables, or text should be explained. Numbers reduced because of incomplete patient data should be clearly reconciled with the number of patients originally enrolled, especially if the reduced numbers appear in tables, figures, or graphs.[9,27–29]

While limited amounts of missing data from incomplete observations of patients can generally be managed, a more serious problem is the lack of data due to patient withdrawal or dropout. Patients who withdraw are often omitted from the figures, graphs, or tables used to illustrate the reported results and are sometimes not included in the data used to evaluate the drug's clinical efficacy and safety. The omission of these types of data may create a misleading impression about the investigational drug's efficacy and safety because the focus would be on the patients who tolerated the drug and not on the complete range of patients in the original target population. Thus, it would be unwise to draw conclusions regarding the value of an investigational drug from the reported results of a trial in which a significant number of patients have withdrawn. Even if omitting data from withdrawn patients will not affect the trial results, the investigators' failure to clearly address the withdrawal problem creates a feeling of uncertainty about the potential bias present in the interpretation of the trial findings.[9,10,30]

## Intention-to-Treat Analysis

The loss of patients or patient data during a clinical drug trial can affect the comparability of the patients in the experimental and control groups, resulting in a misleading interpretation of the efficacy and safety of the investigational drug. Although random assignment ensures that the patients in the experimental and control groups are initially similar, the loss of data due to incomplete record keeping or patient withdrawal could result in the groups being dissimilar at the end of the trial. The most accepted approach to preserving this similarity is called intention-to-treat (ITT) analysis.[12,31]

Intention-to-treat analysis is a conceptual approach to handling missing data or patient withdrawals and is recommended by the Food and Drug Administration (FDA) for clinical drug trials, primarily for phase III and IV studies. This analysis incorporates all enrolled patients regardless of whether they completed the study or had a complete data file. Quite often, the investigator presents two types of analyses, one based on intention to treat and the other not.[12,31]

There appears to be wide acceptance of the necessity to include all patients in the analysis of the investigational drug. There is, however, a disagreement regarding who these patients should be. The choice appears to be based more on the investigator's experience and understanding of good statistical practices in handling incomplete data sets than on any accepted guideline. Various choices include[12,31]

- all patients randomized to the experimental and control groups,

- all patients who were correctly randomized (which would exclude ineligible patients),

- all patients correctly randomized who have had at least one evaluation (this includes only patients who actively participated), or

- all those correctly randomized patients who received at least one dose of the drug (which would include only patients who had actually begun the treatment phase).

Each choice can be justified by the study objectives and may produce different results, depending on the extent of patient withdrawals and missing data.

It is clear that intention-to-treat analysis should be presented in any clinical drug trial with a large number of patient withdrawals or missing data. However, because of the controversy involved in implementation of this approach, investigators often perform at least two sets of analysis, one based on intention-to-treat principles and the other usually based on a subset of patients who have completed the trial or a complete data profile on the outcome of interest. The intention-to-treat analysis would represent a conservative estimate of the investigational drug's effects while the other analysis could be perceived as a more positive assessment. Thus, the healthcare practitioner can consider which estimate is more plausible and applicable to routine practice.[31]

## Interim Analysis

The costs of performing clinical research and the need for innovative new drug therapy has led many sponsors of large-scale, long-term trials to incorporate "data checks" while the study is in progress. This check, based on a preliminary examination of incomplete patient data, is commonly called interim analysis. It examines the preliminary results after breaking the blinding code to identify patients receiving the test drug and those receiving the control.[2]

The decision to perform interim analysis is almost always that of the drug sponsor, although the FDA may request an analysis based on safety. The primary purpose is to make a decision whether or not to stop a clinical drug trial early because of safety issues, lack of clinical efficacy, or, most likely, the expectation that the investigational drug will demonstrate clinical superiority compared to the control treatment. Interim analysis is different from other intermediate analyses done to check on research quality. The latter type of analysis is commonly called administrative analysis and focuses on examining the patient recruitment rate, patient and investigator adherence to the protocol, and the quality of the data collection and management procedures. Unlike in interim analysis, the blind procedure rarely needs to be broken.[32,33]

While preliminary data examination can be justified, it has a significant potential to result in a biased interpretation. Ending prematurely may exaggerate the reported results because of the tendency to stop a trial at the point when the expected differences between the investigational and control drug are greatest. It is possible that the size of the difference is a random occurrence and will decrease if the trial continues. To avoid these problems, the FDA guidelines request that the drug sponsor document in the protocol all planned interim analyses. This documentation should provide a clear rationale for the interim analysis and the planned number of times when the analysis will be performed. The rationale should describe what would be examined (i.e., number of patients who experience the outcome or event rates such as death) and the timing of the analyses. The planned number of times to examine the data should be minimized to preserve the ability to statistically identify true differences at the end. Procedures for maintaining the blind protocol should be described. The stopping rules, criteria used to stop the clinical drug trial, should be clearly specified.[32,33]

Any deviation from these plans may be a serious violation of the study protocol and would cast doubt on its conclusions. Unplanned interim analyses are discouraged because they may introduce bias into the statistical interpretation of the results. Where such unplanned interim analyses are unavoidable, the investigators must clearly document the purpose of the analysis and demonstrate that statistical bias has been minimized.[4,32,33]

Despite the availability of a significant amount of statistical research on how to perform interim analysis, misuse of the practice continues. There seems to be confusion and lack of consensus among investigators regarding what constitutes an interim analysis, when it is necessary to specify a stopping rule, and the statistical implications of such actions. This disagreement has widened because of the use of vaguely defined and misunderstood terms such as "administrative looks," "administrative interim analysis," "interim analysis for safety," and "interim analysis for sample size adjustment." This activity represents a significant potential for biased results.[32]

Nevertheless, interim analysis is an important tool in the development of new drugs, especially for life-threatening or severely debilitating illnesses. Monitoring the trial results as they emerge is particularly important if the results are to positively affect patient survival. An example is the first clinical study of the AIDS drug zidovudine (AZT). Because drug therapy was needed to reduce high mortality rates, interim analyses were included in the protocol. From these analyses, a clear survival advantage for patients receiving zidovudine was observed well before the trial was scheduled to end. The trial was then ended early, and within a week FDA authorized a protocol allowing more than 4000 patients to receive zidovudine before it was approved for marketing.[34]

# References

1. Barnett-Parexel International Training Group. *An Overview of Drug Development.* San Diego: Barnett International; 1998:25–33.

2. Kassalow LM. Statistical and data management: collaboration in clinical research. In: Gaurino RA, ed. *New Drug Approval Process: The Global Challenge.* 3rd ed. New York: Marcel Dekker; 2000:289–310.

3. Pocock SJ. Protocol deviations. In: Pocock SJ, ed. *Clinical Trials: A Practical Approach.* New York: Wiley; 1983:176–86.

4. Gaurino RA. Clinical research protocols. In: Gaurino RA, ed. *New Drug Approval Process: The Global Challenge.* 3rd ed. New York: Marcel Dekker; 2000:219–46.

5. DeMets D. Distinction between fraud, bias, errors, misunderstanding, and incompetence. *Controlled Clin Trials.* 1997; 18:637–50.

6. Groenewoud G, Bell PJ. The need for pre-trial audits in clinical trials-an investigator's perspective. *Drug Info J.* 1995; 29:639–44.

7. Mackintosh DR. Detection of negligence, fraud, and other bad faith efforts during field auditing of clinical trial sites. *Drug Info J.* 1996; 30:645–53.

8. Koch GG, Sollecito WA. Statistical considerations in the design, analysis and interpretation of comparative clinical studies. *Drug Info J.* 1984; 18:131–51.

9. Bailar JC, Mosteller F. Guidelines for statistical reporting in articles for medical journals. In: Bailar JC, Mosteller F, eds. *Medical Use of Statistics.* Boston: NEJM Books; 1992:313–31.

10. Kirwin JR. Clinical trials: why not do them properly? *Ann Rheum Dis.* 1982; 41:551–2.

11. Elwood MJ. *Critical Appraisal of Epidemiological Studies and Clinical Trials.* New York: Oxford University Press; 1998:116–60.

12. Svensson K. How many populations must be analyzed and how should they be defined (intent-to-treat, eligible, per protocol population, etc.)? *Drug Info J.* 1995; 29(2):475–8.

13. Vrijens B, Goetghebeur E. The impact of compliance in pharmacokinetic studies. *Stat Methods Med Res.* 1999; 8:247–62.

14. Kramer MS, Shapiro SH. Scientific challenges in the application of randomized trials. *JAMA.* 1984; 252:2739–45.

15. Freedman LS. The effect of partial non-compliance on the power of a clinical trial. *Controlled Clin Trials.* 1990; 11:157–68.

16. Lasagna L. Balancing risks versus benefits in drug therapy decisions. *Clin Ther.* 1998; 20:C72–C79.

17. Hagen E, Istad H, Ose L, et al. Fluvastatin efficacy and tolerability in comparison and in combination with cholestyramine. *Eur J Clin Pharmacol.* 1994; 46:445–9.

18. Hunninghake DB, Stein EA, Dujovne CA, et al. The efficacy of intensive dietary therapy alone or combined with lovastatin in outpatients with hypercholesterolemia. *N Engl J Med.* 1993; 328:1213–9.

19. Subcutaneous Sumatriptan Study Group. Treatment of migraine attacks with sumatriptan. *N Engl J Med.* 1991; 325:316–21.

20. McGuire WP, Hoskins WJ, Brady MF, et al. Cyclophosphamide and cisplatin compared with paclitaxel and cisplatin in patients with stage III and stage IV ovarian cancer. *N Engl J Med.* 1996; 334:1–6.

21. United States Pharmacopeia. *Drug Information for the Health Professional.* 20th ed. Rockville MD: United States Pharmacopeial Convention, Inc.; 2000

22. Berzon RA. Understanding and using health-related quality of life instruments within clinical research studies. In: Staquet MJ, Hays RD, Fayers PM, eds. *Quality of Life Assessment in Clinical Trials.* New York: Oxford University Press; 1998:3–15.

23. Polk RE, Hepler CD. Controversies in antimicrobial therapy: critical analysis of clinical trials. *Am J Hosp Pharm.* 1986; 43:630–40.

24. Moscucci M, Byrne L, Weintraub M, et al. Blinding, unblinding, and the placebo effect: an analysis of patients' guesses of treatment assignment in a double-blind clinical trial. *Clin Pharmacol Ther.* 1987; 41:259–65.

25. Pocock SJ. *Clinical Trials: A Practical Approach.* New York: Wiley; 1983:111.

26. Hallstrom A, Davis K. Imbalance in treatment assignments in stratified blocked randomization. *Controlled Clin Trials.* 1988; 9:375–82.

27. Walker AM. Reporting the results of epidemiologic studies. *Am J Pub Health.* 1986; 76:556–8.

28. Moses LE. Statistical concepts fundamental to investigations. In: Bailar JC, Mosteller F, eds. *Medical Use of Statistics.* Boston: NEJM Books; 1992:5–25.

29. Hamilton CW. How to write and publish scientific papers: scribing information for pharmacists. *Am J Hosp Pharm.* 1992; 49:2477–84.

30. Barnes RW. Understanding investigative clinical trials. *J Vasc Surg.* 1989; 9:609–18.

31. Unnebrink K, Windeler J. Sensitivity analysis by worst and best case assessment: is it really sensitive? *Drug Info J.* 1999; 33:835–9.

32. Sankoh AJ. Interim analysis: An update of an FDA reviewer's experience and perspectives. *Drug Info J.* 1999; 33:165–76.

33. Leroy A, Buyse M, Harrison M, et al. Interim analysis. *Drug Info J.* 1995; 29:507–8.

34. FDA Center for Drug Evaluation and Research. *From Test Tube to Patient: Improving Health Through Human Drugs.* Rockville MD: Food and Drug Administration; 1999:18–23.

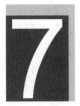

# Results:
# Presentation of Data

□

➤□ 18. Are descriptive statistics used properly to describe the trial results?

➤□ 19. How accurate and complete are the tables, figures, and graphs?

□

In addition to a discussion of trial management, the results section of an article includes the study findings describing what actually occurred. Most information is quantitative, with an emphasis on the presentation of numbers through the use of descriptive statistics such as the mean, standard deviation, confidence interval, Pearson product moment correlation, or incidence rates. These statistics are provided throughout the text and in tables, figures, and graphs.

Descriptive statistics, if used properly, provide an unbiased view of the study results. The reported data should be self-explanatory and generally free of the investigators' interpretation. When presented results are confusing, it may suggest a poorly managed data collection system, lack of clear study objectives, poor study design, or intentional investigator bias.

This chapter describes the type of statistics that should be used in the results section to effectively summarize the findings of the clinical drug trial (Question 18). The discussion includes a description of the statistic, how it should be used, and how to assess its appropriateness for the clinical drug trial described. The second part of the chapter (Question 19) describes visual tools (e.g., figures, graphs, or tables) used to present data effectively. Different tools are discussed along with a description of their purpose and use.

# ☑ 18. Are descriptive statistics used properly to describe the trial results?

After the raw data are collected, they should be organized into a usable form, and the characteristics of patients and their responses should be numerically described. This process is often referred to as descriptive statistics and provides a convenient, effective method for the investigator to describe the results. The use of descriptive statistics depends on the purpose of the clinical drug trial and the preferences of the investigator and may vary from trial to trial. Some uses are described in Table 7-1. Regardless of the approach, the potential for misleading use of the descriptive statistic always exists. A flawed approach to describing the data results in inappropriate conclusions and misleading theories about the data collected.[1–4]

**Table 7-1** Selected Use of Descriptive Statistics

| Purpose | Description |
| --- | --- |
| **Quantifying responses** | Quantifying patient responses into continuous or discrete data for later statistical analysis or interpretation |
| **Assessing data distribution** | Examining whether the data are arranged in a normal distribution through the use of frequency distributions, histograms, or scatter diagrams |
| **Measuring centrality** | Describing the central part of the data with measures such as the mean, median, or mode |
| **Measuring variability** | Estimating the spread of the data through the use of measures such as the range or standard deviation |
| **Estimating the target population** | Using the confidence interval to describe the group mean and response rates of the target population in which the study sample was derived |
| **Examining relationships** | Using correlational analysis and linear regression to examine relationships between two or more measures |
| **Assessing important rare events** | Using the incidence and prevalence rates to determine the safety profile of an investigational drug |

## Quantifying Responses

Patient responses usually are converted into numbers for interpretation and analysis. Quite often, the initial conversion is done when the measurement instrument is created and used. Even if patient responses are converted to numerical data at the time of measurement, further categorization is often done when the raw data are organized and analyzed.

This categorization is generally not standardized and depends on the purpose of the study and the experience and perspective of the investigator.[5]

Patient responses to measures are usually converted into numerical data called variables. Variables are the measured numerical values obtained from patient responses and can vary from one measurement to another. These variables can be either discrete or continuous.[6-9]

Discrete (or categorical) variables have a limited number of values (or data scales) that should not overlap. Those variables that include responses that can be named (e.g., success or failure of a treatment) are often called nominal variables, while variables with responses that can be numerically ordered (e.g., degree of pain reported) are called ordinal.

Conversely, continuously scaled variables may include an infinite number of evenly spaced values, usually restricted only by the upper and lower limits of the instrument used. The responses are generally classified into interval and ratio scales, although in practice the distinction between the two scales is often unclear because instruments generally measure a finite range of data (Table 7-2).[6-9]

While the distinction between the discrete and continuous variables is theoretically clear, in practice the two types of variables are used interchangeably. Discrete variables that are ordinally scaled are often analyzed by statistics designed for continuous variables. The statistical argument to justify this use is that ordinally scaled data, like responses with interval or ratio scales, may have a distinct order of magnitude and equal gaps between the scales. In addition, continuous data can be classified into discrete variables with nominal or ordinal scales.[6-9]

While the definition of variables used to describe the collected data is standardized and often based on the type of measuring instrument, the way in which investigators use the scales varies. The choice of method may greatly affect the interpretation of the results. If an investigator converts continuous variables into discrete categories, valuable data may be lost. Any reclassification of the data should clearly distinguish between the different categories.[1,10] An example would be the data collected to assess the efficacy of an investigational antihypertensive drug. The primary outcome assessed may be "blood pressure control," as measured by changes in the blood pressure. Although blood pressure is measured on a continuous scale, investigators often divide the patients into subgroups who are "controlled" and "not controlled," with the former consisting of patients with a diastolic pressure lower than 95 mm Hg on the sphygmomanometer. The investigator would report a percentage of patients who achieve the desired goal, but the results may be misleading. Some patients classified as "controlled" may have a diastolic blood pressure as high as 94 mm Hg. That value is not very different from the minimum value of 95 mm Hg needed to classify a patient as "not controlled."

**Table 7-2** Classification of Data Scales[1,8]

| Classification | Description |
| --- | --- |
| **Nominal** | The least complicated scale and weakest level of measurement. Data are classified by an assigned number in which patients are placed in subgroups based on similar characteristics. Nominal scales are used to describe two or more groups of patients. Examples would include assigning numerical categories that designate patients as male or female, cured or not cured, or receiving the investigational or control drug. The numbers selected to describe each group are arbitrary and are usually chosen at the discretion of the investigator (i.e., 1 = male 2 = female).There cannot be any overlap among the groups. |
| **Ordinal** | The data are ranked in a specific order, usually low to high. A typical ordinal scale would rank the amount of ankle swelling from "one" (very little or none) to "three" (a great deal). The numbers chosen are scored on a continuum, although the level of difference between different sets of numbers may not be consistent. The actual number assigned is not important as long as the different evaluators consistently assign higher (or lower) numbers to the relatively more important subgroup. |
| **Interval** | The scales are based on predetermined numbering like ordinal scales but also include a consistent difference between each number. The scale lacks a true "zero point" that would indicate no data present. An example would be a measure of the patient's age. |
| **Ratio** | Similar to the interval scale except that there is a true zero point. Heart rate, blood pressure, and time to demonstrate an effect are examples of ratio scales. |

The type of data scales created influences the choice of statistical tests used and their effectiveness in detecting differences between the experimental and control groups. The more powerful statistical tests should be used only with continuously scaled data. In addition, loss of information with the use of discrete scales makes any statistical test less sensitive in identifying true differences between the experimental and control groups.[1,8–11]

## Assessing Data Distribution

Examination of the distribution of any data set is based on the principle that the data are a sample for the total population of values. The extent that these data represent the larger target population is important for generalizing the results. Thus, it is helpful if the investigator addresses the distribution or "shape" of the data for potential generalizability. In addition, many statistical tests are based on assumptions about the data distribution.

### Normal distribution

The desired shape for continuous data is the normal distribution.[4,6,7,12–15] The normal distribution of data points is the most common and means that the data are symmetrically scattered around a central point. Its value is based on the central limit theorem, which states that the distribution of data points from a sufficiently large sample will always be close to a normal distribution. There is no specific sample size required for this theorem to be valid. However, sample sizes as small as 30 may approximate this distribution. The central limit theorem is critical to the use of statistics because it justifies the assumption of the normal distribution needed for many calculations.

The shape of this distribution is often referred to as a "bell-shaped" curve. The curve is also called a Gaussian, normal distribution, or normal probability curve (Figure 7-1). The term bell-shaped is a misnomer because many bell-shaped curves have different peaks or spreads. Nevertheless, the term traditionally is applied to a normally distributed set of values.

**Figure 7-1** Normal Distribution Curve

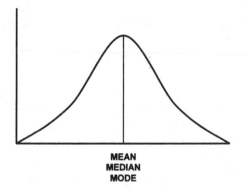

**MEAN**
**MEDIAN**
**MODE**

An infinite number of normal distributions are possible for target populations studied in clinical drug trials. The shape of these distributions depends on the mean score for the population and the degree of variability. To make this distribution more understandable and useful, investigators often convert the range of numbers to a standard normal curve. Statistically, the curve's features define the standard normal distribution: it has a mean of zero and a standard deviation and variance of one and the tails of the distribution extend from minus infinity to positive infinity.

A major use of the standard normal distribution is to convert raw data scores into standard units to show the relative position of that score in the distribution. Understanding the value of a patient data score of 100 on a clinical outcome measure would be difficult unless the relative meaning of the score was known. The relative position of the score is learned by converting it into a standardized score known as a z score. Statistically, the z score expresses the distance of the patient score from the mean of the target population using the standard deviation as the standard distance measure. The z score indicates how many standard deviations the patient score is away from the mean. This standardized transformation does not alter the form of the raw distribution of numbers in the sample. The frequency of each patient score in the sample remains the same regardless of whether the distribution is standardized or not.

The conversion of raw data into a standard normal curve makes the interpretation of statistical tests more useful. In addition, investigators can make comparisons between data sets that may be on different scales or have different values. Thus, differences between the data sets may be more easily detected and understood.

### Other distributions for continuous data

In addition to normal distribution, continuous data are sometimes arranged into statistically less desirable shapes. Two common arrangements in a clinical drug trial are bimodal and skewed distribution curves.[6,9,16] Bimodal distributions occur when the data are clustered around two distinctly high points in the curve (Figure 7-2). An example would be the bimodal concentration peaks of patients who metabolize a drug differently (slow and fast metabolizers). Although less common, the distribution is considered multimodal if more than two distinct peaks occur.

**Figure 7-2** Bimodal Distribution

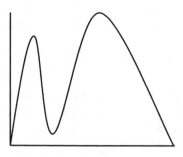

Skewed data curves occur when the data are distributed asymmetrically with one side of the curve extending out in an elongated fashion (Figure 7-3). The curve length of one section is proportionally longer than the other. This distribution is considered positively skewed if the data curve is longer on the right of the high point and negatively skewed if longer on the left. An example of a skewed distribution would be the delayed response to a slow-acting tricyclic antidepressant (negative skew).

**Figure 7-3** Skewed Distribution

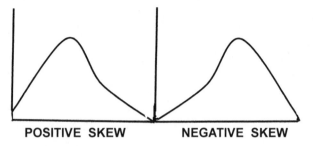

**POSITIVE SKEW**          **NEGATIVE SKEW**

One of the easiest ways to examine normality is to prepare a table of frequency distributions that organizes the data into discrete intervals (Table 7-3). Methods vary for presenting frequency distributions in tables. Nevertheless, the intervals chosen should reflect the data collected, and empty intervals or those with small numbers should be avoided. The number of intervals should be sufficient to clearly describe the data, but an excessive number is undesirable.[6]

**Table 7-3**   An Example Table of Frequency Distribution: Serum Cholesterol Changes for 156 Patients after Administration of a Cholesterol-Lowering Drug [a]

| Interval (mg %)[b] | Frequency (patients) |
| --- | --- |
| −100 to −81 | 1 |
| − 80 to −61 | 6 |
| − 60 to −41 | 16 |
| − 40 to −21 | 31 |
| − 20 to − 1 | 40 |
| 0 to +19 | 43 |
| + 20 to +39 | 16 |
| + 40 to +59 | 3 |

[a] Adapted with permission from Table 1.2 in Bolton S. *Pharmaceutical Statistics*. 2nd ed. New York: Marcel Dekker; 1990:6.
[b] Represents the change from baseline in serum cholesterol after the cholesterol-lowering drug was administered.

Another approach presents data as cumulative frequencies used to quickly demonstrate the cumulative effect of the investigational drug (Table 7-4). Like Table 7-3, the type and number of intervals used should be carefully selected.[6]

**Table 7-4**    An Example Table of Cumulative Frequency Distributions:
Serum Cholesterol Changes for 156 Patients after Administration of
a Cholesterol-Lowering Drug [a]

| Interval (mg %)[b] | Cumulative Frequency (patients) | Cumulative Proportion |
|---|---|---|
| −100 to −81 | 1 | 0.01 |
| − 80 to −61 | 7 | 0.04 |
| − 60 to −41 | 23 | 0.15 |
| − 40 to −21 | 54 | 0.35 |
| − 20 to − 1 | 94 | 0.60 |
| 0 to +19 | 137 | 0.88 |
| +20 to +39 | 153 | 0.98 |
| +40 to +59 | 156 | 1.00 |

[a] Adapted with permission from Table 1.2 in Bolton S. *Pharmaceutical Statistics*. 2nd ed. New York: Marcel Dekker; 1990:6.
[b] Represents the change from baseline in serum cholesterol after the cholesterol-lowering drug was administered.

Histograms and scatter diagrams graphically illustrate data distribution. Histograms are graphic representations of the frequency tables and, like the tables, their value depends on the types of intervals (Figure 7-4). Scatter diagrams show the relationship between two continuously scaled measures (Figure 7-5). Histograms or scatter diagrams may provide better visual displays of data distribution than tables but lack the detail of the tabular method.[6,17,18]

**Figure 7-4**    Sample Histogram Showing the Serum Cholesterol Changes for 156
Patients after Administration of a Cholesterol-Lowering Drug[a,b]

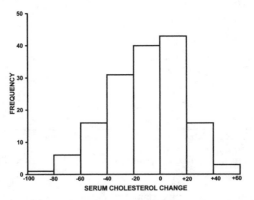

[a]   The horizontal axis represents the change from baseline in serum cholestrol after the cholesterol-lowering drug is administered. The vertical represents the number of patients in each interval.
[b]   Adapted with permission from Figure 2.7 in Bolton S. *Pharmaceutical Statistics*, 2nd ed. New York: Marcel Dekker, 1990:37.

**Figure 7-5** Sample Scatter Diagram Showing the Relationship between Serum Immunoglobulin E (IgE) and Age[a]

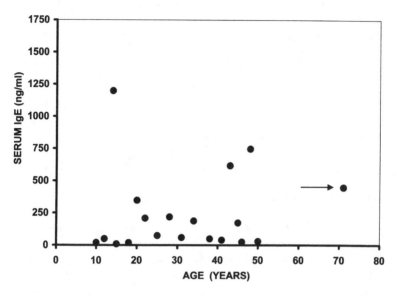

[a]Adapted with permission from Figure 3.1 in O'Brien PC, Shampo MA. *Statistics for Clinicians: 3. Graphic displays-scatter diagrams. Mayo Clin Proc.* 1981;56:196–7.

Besides tabular or graphic analysis of the data distribution, the investigator can measure shape by assessing the degree of skewness or kurtosis of the data. Skewness is the measure of symmetry of a curve. Kurtosis refers to shape of the distribution.[9]

### Binomial distributions

Continuous variables may be arranged in various frequency distributions. However, for discrete variables, the possible values are limited to the number of categories used. The distribution of these values is based on the probability of a patient's response occurring in one category. Thus, most distributions of discrete variables are called probability curves. One commonly occurring probability curve is the binomial distribution.[6,9,16]

The binomial distribution consists of two mutually exclusive outcomes such as the success or failure of an antibiotic to cure a urinary tract infection (Figure 7-6). The data are discrete (cure/no cure) and independent of each other (patient cannot be cured and not cured after treatment). The distribution is based on the probability of an outcome and the number of trials or measurements. A derivation of the binomial distribution is the Poisson distribution. The Poisson distribution is applied when one of the two possible results (such as the presence of a rare side effect) is relatively small.[6,9,16]

**Figure 7-6** Binomial Distribution

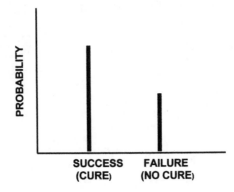

## Measuring Centrality

Measures of centrality or central tendency include the mean, median, and mode and measure the central part of the data.[6,7,13,15,19] The most common measure of centrality is the mean, which is the arithmetic average of the data values. The mean is most effective for normally distributed data that are ratio or intervally scaled. The measure is less effective for ordinally scaled data and is of little value for data nominally scaled. The accuracy of the mean is distorted when extreme values, known as outliers, are present. The mean is also more likely to be distorted if there are relatively few patients.

The median is the middle value (the 50th percentile) of a data set. Thus, half the data points are less than the median and half are greater. Unlike the mean, the median is unaffected by outliers and may be better for data not normally distributed. The median is a better measure than the mean for ordinally scaled data but, like the mean, is not useful for nominally scaled data.

The mode is the value that occurs most frequently in the data. The mode is used less often than the mean or median and is useful with data clustered around two high points (bimodal curve) or one relatively high peak. However, the mode is less useful than other measures of centrality in data generated from small numbers of patients. Unlike the mean and median, the mode can describe nominally scaled data.

While measures of centrality tend to be effective even if some assumptions regarding the distribution or the scaling of the data are violated, the choice of which measures to use should be based on a clear understanding of how the data are distributed. Although the mean, median, and mode represent the same value when the data are normally distributed (Figure 7-1), they are no longer interchangeable when the data distributions become skewed or bimodal (Figures 7-2 and 7-3). Thus, use of the wrong descriptive statistic results in a misleading assessment of the data and a distorted impression of the effectiveness of the investigational drug.[6,7,13,19]

## Measuring Variability

Measuring the variability of data is important because it estimates the value of the measure of centrality.[1,6-8,10,12,13,15,16,19-21] It is not useful for discrete variables nominally scaled because there is no real measure of centrality. Assessing the variability of a measure of continuously or ordinally scaled variables gives insight into how close the measure of centrality (most often the mean) is to representing the group scores of the patients. For example, data points widely scattered from the mean give a different perspective than data points very close to the mean.

Common measures of variability are the range, percentile, and standard deviation. These measures determine how closely individual patient values cluster around the center part of the data. A large variability in the data suggests the presence of a flaw in the trial design: unreliable measures may have been used, the subjects selected may not be very similar, or the data collected may not be normally distributed. The last problem would make the use of many descriptive statistics and tests of significance less appropriate (*see* Chapter 8, Question 20).[6,7,13,15]

The range is the difference between the smallest and largest value in the data set. Although easy to understand, the range has limited use because it is strongly influenced by the most extreme values in the data and tends to be affected by the number of patients, increasing with sample size. The range should be used only as a rough measure of the variability.[6,7,13,15]

Percentiles are measures of variability based on the median value, which would be considered the 50th percentile of the range of data in a clinical drug trial. The most likely use of percentiles is through the use of the interquartile range, which is the interval between the data score at the first quartile (25th percentile) and the third quartile (75th percentile). The interquartile range is used to get a rough impression of the middle 50% of the data and has an advantage over other measures of variability because it is less dependent on the number of patients. Another advantage is that the assumption of a normal distribution is not needed.[6,7,13,15]

The standard deviation (SD) is the most commonly used measure of variability, assuming a standardized normal distribution. If all patient data scores were the same as the group mean, the standard deviation would be zero. Conversely, the standard deviation increases as the patient data scores are farther from the group mean. The standard deviation is commonly expressed as the "mean +/- SD." The utility of the standard deviation is based on its ability to define data distribution more accurately than the other measures of variability. Assuming that the data are distributed normally, it is expected that 68.2% of the data scores would lie one standard deviation on either side of the mean and 95.4% of the scores would occur within two standard deviations. Almost all values (99.7%) would be within three standard deviations of the mean (Figure 7-7). For example, if the mean maximum concentration at four hours of an 800-mg dose of the anticonvulsant drug felbamate is 14.3 +/− 1.4 µg/ml, then 68.2% of the patients have values from 12.9 to 15.7 µg/ml, 95.4% have concentrations from 11.5 to 17.1 µg/ml, and 99.7% have concentrations from 10.1 to 18.5 µg/ml. [1,7,13,15,16,20]

A measure closely related to the standard deviation is the variance, a more general measure of data spread. The variance is the square of the standard deviation. Thus, the variance of the serum felbamate concentration was 1.96 µg/ml. The standard deviation is often preferred over the variance because it is generally more understandable and can more easily identify data dispersion. [1,7,13,15,16,20]

**Figure 7-7** Use of Standard Deviations to Estimate Spread in a Normal Distribution[a]

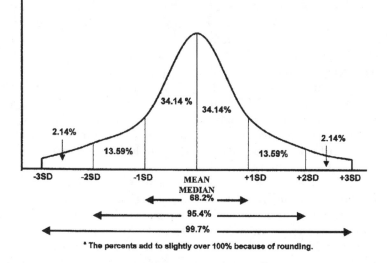

ᵃ The percents add to slightly over 100% because of rounding.

In comparing two groups with equal means, the standard deviation gives an idea of how many individuals in each group were scattered from the mean and thus estimates the appropriateness of the mean score. Investigators should always report the standard deviation when presenting the mean score so that the reader gets a sense of the data variability. For example, a large variability in the mean score of a primary outcome measure indicates that some patients are responding much better than others within the study group. [1,7,13,15,16,20]

A measure often confused with the standard deviation is the standard error of the mean or SEM. This measure is sometimes called the standard deviation of the mean or the standard error. The standard deviation describes the variability within a sample, while the standard error of the mean represents the possible variability of the mean itself. [1,6,8,10,13,21]

The standard error of the mean is based on the premise that each sample obtained from the target population would have a group mean that differs from the "true" or population mean. The SEM measures the degree of variation that occurs each time that a patient sample is obtained. Less variation suggests that each group sample mean obtained is close to the population mean and would produce more applicable results.[1,6,8,10,13,21]

The SEM is derived from the standard deviation (it equals the standard deviation of the sample data divided by the square root of the sample size) and is always smaller, which sometimes results in misleading use of the statistic. Authors may erroneously use the SEM to represent the level of data dispersion around the mean, but this use would be misleading because it has a different meaning than the standard deviation. The SEM is smaller and its use instead of the larger standard deviation may be a biased manipulation intended to make data look more reliable.[1,6,8,10,13,21]

The SEM is extremely important in estimating characteristics of the target population that eventually uses the drug. However, because it is disproportionately low, it should never be used as a measure dispersion of the patient sample results.[1,6,8,10,13,21]

## Estimating the Target Population

One purpose of descriptive statistics is to statistically characterize the population from which the sample was derived. In clinical drug trials, the descriptive statistics usually estimate the mean score and drug response rates that typically occur in the target population.[6,8,9,13,16,22,23] This approach is used to determine the possible range of scores expected if the investigational drug were tested on multiple samples of the same population. This information is critical for comparing the effects of the investigational drug and the control treatment (*see* Chapter 8, Question 20) and also for assessing reliability and validity.

An example would be the hypothetical reporting of the diastolic blood pressure readings of patients in a clinical trial of a new antihypertensive drug. The patients in the experimental group had an average diastolic blood pressure reading of 92.2 mm Hg, while the diastolic blood pressure of the group receiving the control treatments was 95.1 mm Hg. These scores are averages derived from patients selected from the whole population of patients suffering from hypertension. Because it is a sample, the investigator would not be sure that the same results would occur if the investigational drug were administered to another sample of the same population. To generalize the results to the target population using the drug in practice, the investigator estimates the probable range of scores expected if another sample were exposed to the investigational drug under the same conditions.

An effective tool for this estimation is the confidence interval. Confidence intervals (CIs) find the "true" score of a statistic by estimating the range of scores in which the true value is likely to occur.[6,9,16,22]

Confidence limits represent the upper and lower extent of the confidence interval. The accepted width of the confidence interval depends on data variability and an arbitrarily chosen degree of confidence, traditionally 95%. A CI of 95% implies that if a study were conducted 100 times, the value found would fall within the CI 95 times. Like the standard deviation, the confidence interval can be expressed as the mean $+/-$ the standard error. Usually the CI term is added to avoid confusion. More likely, however, the CI is expressed as a range of values. Thus, the hypothetical standard deviation of the experimental group sample's diastolic blood pressure readings may be 92.2 $+/-$ 3.4 SD, and the confidence interval may be expressed as (95% CI, 84.8–99.6 mm Hg). Thus, the investigator is 95% confident that the estimated "true" mean diastolic blood pressure for the target population is between 84.8 and 99.6 mg Hg. Expanding the confidence interval increases the likelihood of predicting the correct population mean. However, a very large confidence interval makes estimation of the actual mean difficult. In all cases, the estimation assumes that the sample data truly reflect the same statistical characteristics of the target population. A study sample with a severely skewed distribution of data points would likely produce a CI that does not include the population mean.

Confidence intervals describe many outcomes of a clinical drug trial but are particularly useful in the description of drug safety. On a quantitative measure of toxicity (such as liver function), the use of the confidence interval provides the information about the upper and lower limits of the average score for the study groups. This information would be helpful if there is a preestablished safety level. If the range is below the safety level, the investigational drug could be considered safe. A range that goes beyond this level may make the drug appear to be more toxic.[23]

## Examining Relationships

Investigators often quantify and explore the strength of relationships between various variables. The most common applications are for

- defining and characterizing the investigational drug's dose–response relationships,

- establishing its pharmacokinetic and pharmacodynamic profile, and

- minimizing the influence of other factors on the efficacy and safety measures used.

Two common methods used for assessing relationships are correlational analysis and linear regression.[1,6,14,24–26]

Correlational analysis evaluates the strength and direction of a relationship between two or more measures. An example is the relationship between the patient's age, weight, or height and the investigational drug's serum level. The measures most often used in correlational analysis are the Pearson product moment correlation and Spearman rank order correlation, which are represented by the notation r. Pearson or Spearman r values range from 0 (no association) to 1 (complete agreement). A minus sign is usually attached when the relationship is negative (i.e., going in an opposite direction). Because complete agreement between two measures is rare, the importance of any relationship is usually based on the subjective opinion of the investigators. Nevertheless, a relationship with an r value of 0.88 (normally reported as r = 0.88) between the patient's age and the investigational drug's serum level would generally be considered strong while an r value of 0.12 (reported as r = 0.12) would usually be considered weak. Correlational analysis should be limited only to the exploration of possible relationships among the measures present in the clinical drug trial because it tends to identify associations that are arbitrary and ambiguous. It should not be used to establish causal relationships[1,14,24,25] (*see* Chapter 9, Question 22).

Linear regression describes the relationship between multiple measures by finding the best fitting straight line among the data collected. Mathematically, linear regression examines the rate of change in one measure related to a change in another and is expressed by

$$y = a + bx + e$$

where *y* represents one measure and *x* is the other; *a* is the *y*-intercept or the point on the *y*-axis where the regression lines cross (the value of *y* when *x* = 0), *b* is the slope or the amount of change in *y* for every unit increase in *x*, and *e* is the term for the random error present in the data. The random error term is often eliminated from the equation before publication.[1,6,24,26]

Simple linear regression examines the relationship between two measures, and multiple linear regression explores the association among more than two measures. The regression line is usually calculated with the least-squares method, designed to find where the line comes closest to running through all data points (best fit). The most commonly used measure of the effectiveness of the linear regression line is the coefficient of determination, represented by the notation $r^2$. The $r^2$ is equal to 1 when all data points are on the regression line and is equal to 0 when there is no linear relationship among the data. Like the r term in correlational analysis, the $r^2$ is rarely equal to 1. Thus, the importance of the $r^2$ of any linear regression is based on the investigator's subjective opinion. Linear regression, like correlational analysis, should be limited to examining associations among the various measures in the clinical drug trial but should not be used as the sole basis for establishing a causal relationship between two or more measures.[1,6,24,26]

## Assessing Important Events

The measures of centrality and variability are used to assess the impact of the investigational drug. These descriptive statistics describe expected, common events such as symptom relief or cure of the disease being studied. However, the statistics are limited when the incidence of the expected outcome is relatively rare.[22,23,27] An example would be the identification of infrequently occurring and often unpredictable adverse drug events (ADEs). Each of these events is important, especially if it significantly harms a patient. Because most clinical phase II and III drug trials primarily establish the investigational drug's efficacy, rare or infrequent events may go undetected. Detecting such events is often the focus of phase IV clinical trials, especially those that involve postmarketing surveillance.

In both types of designs, descriptive statistics such as the mean, standard deviation, and confidence interval are limited when summarizing the data about ADEs, because their occurrence is not normally distributed. Thus, a more suitable set of measures would be the incidence and prevalence rates, typically associated with epidemiological or case-control studies.[22,23,27]

The incidence rate measures how many new patients exposed to the investigational drug will develop a specific ADE. The specific formula is:

incidence rate =
$$\frac{\text{number of new patients who experience an ADE}}{\text{total number of patients who participated}}$$

Conversely, the prevalence rate measures the number of patients who have the ADE at any given time, regardless of whether it was a new experience or not. Otherwise, it is the same formula as incidence rate.

prevalence rate =
$$\frac{\text{number of new patients who experience an ADE at a specific time}}{\text{total number of patients who participated up to that time}}$$

The two rates traditionally provide different information. The incidence reflects the rate of occurrence of the ADE while the prevalence reflects all existing cases reported in the trial, regardless of whether they are newly discovered. Incidence rates of ADEs are influenced by many factors, such as when the investigational drug was administered, the presence of other drugs in the regimen, or the cumulative dosing effect of the investigational drug. Prevalence rates are dependent on both the incidence of the ADE and its duration. Thus, short duration ADEs may be missed in a prevalence assessment, while long duration events may not.

How the incidence and prevalence rates of ADEs in a clinical drug trial are used and reported may affect the interpretation of drug safety. If relatively infrequent measurements of safety are used, both the incidence and prevalence of ADEs may be underreported, especially if the ADE has a short-term effect.

The timing of the measures and the duration of the clinical drug trial are also important. Drug safety measured only at the end may miss valuable information about when the ADE actually occurred and thus alter the incidence rate.

However, a longer study likely increases the probability of a rare ADE occurring, and measuring safety at the end will probably result in an increase in its prevalence rate. Both the incidence and prevalence of an ADE should be reported in a manner useful to the healthcare practitioner, such as the incidence (or prevalence) per 1000 patients exposed to the drug.

## ☑ 19. How accurate and complete are the tables, figures, and graphs?

One of the most important objectives of the analysis section is to present the data clearly and concisely through the reporting of relevant statistics in the text, tables, figures, and graphs. Because there are no uniform guidelines on how to present data, the approaches vary, depending on the preferences of the investigator or the publisher. Some investigators prefer to present results graphically, while others favor the greater detail of tables or text. Similar variations in preference occur with journal editors.[2,20,28]

Regardless of the technique used, the number of figures, graphs, and tables should be restricted to that sufficient to complement each other and the text in explaining results and supporting the investigator's observations and conclusions. Too many figures, graphs, and tables unnecessarily fragment the analysis and create clutter. Redundancy should be avoided, and the data should be consistent no matter how and where presented.[2,20,28]

### Use of Tables

Tables present numerical data that might otherwise require several long and awkward sentences. They should be self-explanatory and accurate. The table title should clearly reflect what is contained, and the information included should be comprehensive. Tables are very effective for showing numbers, if done properly.[2,28–30] Although no standards exist, some useful guidelines are shown in Table 7-5.

Tables 7-6 and 7-7 illustrate how the guidelines can be applied to make a table easier to read. The tables compare the death rates

**Table 7-5** Techniques for Displaying Numbers in Tables[2,30]

| Techniques | Description |
| --- | --- |
| **Use of digits** | Use as few as possible (0.11 rather than 0.1105) |
| **Columns and rows** | Present vertically in columns rather than horizontally in rows |
| **Margins** | Margin and row averages should be reported |
| **Order** | Place in consistent, logical order, such as in decreasing or increasing importance |
| **Clarity** | Use layout to ensure clarity and to make information presented self-explanatory |
| **Summaries** | Text summaries of the tables should be brief and focus on the main points of the tables |

observed in four groups in which anesthetics were used in surgeries with high death rates.

Data presentation in Table 7-6 ignores the guidelines presented in Table 7-5 and appears cluttered and difficult to read. The use of five-digit figures and the horizontal presentation of important categories confuse the reader.

**Table 7-6** An Example Table That Lacks Clarity: Death Rates in Proportions for High Death Rate Operations by Anesthetic Risk Levels [a]

| Anesthetic Risk Code | Halothane | Nitrous Oxide | Cyclo-propane | Ether | Other |
| --- | --- | --- | --- | --- | --- |
| Unknown | 0.11369 | 0.08682 | 0.08147 | 0.06148 | 0.09957 |
| Risk 1 | 0.02454 | 0.02452 | 0.01634 | 0.01355 | 0.03358 |
| Risk 2 | 0.05471 | 0.06893 | 0.04941 | 0.03812 | 0.05859 |
| Risk 3 | 0.12471 | 0.16599 | 0.18187 | 0.11453 | 0.15306 |
| Risk 4 | 0.15892 | 0.23140 | 0.18582 | 0.17919 | 0.35531 |
| Risk 5 | 0.04665 | 0.06759 | 0.05725 | 0.04898 | 0.07606 |
| Risk 6 | 0.22143 | 0.12996 | 0.17615 | 0.16008 | 0.17741 |
| Risk 7 | 0.44164 | 0.43689 | 0.36689 | 0.62121 | 0.43348 |

[a] Adapted with permission from Table 1 in Bailar JC, Mosteller F. Guidelines for statistical reporting in articles for medical journals. In: Bailar JC, Mosteller F, eds. *Medical Use of Statistics*. Boston: NEJM Books; 1992:325.

**Table 7-7** An Example Table Based on Clarity Guidelines: Death Rates in Percentages for High Death Rate Operations by Anesthetic Risk Levels versus Anesthetic Risk[a]

| | Anesthetic Risk Code | | | | | | | | |
| Anesthetic | 1 | 2 | 5 | UNK[b] | 3 | 6 | 4 | 7 | WA[b] |
|---|---|---|---|---|---|---|---|---|---|
| Other | 3 | 6 | 8 | 10 | 15 | 18 | 36 | 43 | 11.7 |
| Nitrous oxide | 2 | 7 | 7 | 9 | 17 | 13 | 23 | 44 | 10.3 |
| Cyclopropane | 2 | 5 | 6 | 8 | 18 | 18 | 19 | 37 | 9.8 |
| Halothane | 2 | 5 | 5 | 11 | 12 | 22 | 16 | 44 | 8.7 |
| Ether | 1 | 4 | 5 | 6 | 11 | 16 | 18 | 62 | 6.1 |
| WA[b] | 2.2 | 5.5 | 5.7 | 9.6 | 14.6 | 17.4 | 20.6 | 42.4 | 9.3 |

[a] Adapted with permission from Table 2 in Bailar JC, Mosteller F. Guidelines for statistical reporting in articles for medical journals. In: Bailar JC, Mosteller F, eds. *Medical Use of Statistics*. Boston: NEJM Books; 1992:327.
[b] UNK = unknown; WA = weighted average

Table 7-7 illustrates the results organized according to the Table 7-5 guidelines. The number of digits has been reduced to one or two, the major categories of numbers are presented vertically, marginal and row averages are provided, and the order is based on the weighted average in the last column. Table 7-7 should be summarized in the following manner in the text:[14]

> *The table shows that the overall weighted percentage of deaths in these high death rate operations is 9.3%. When the risk levels are arranged according to the average death rate for the risk, each anesthetic leads to a nearly monotonic increase in death rate according to risk, the order being codes 1,2,5, unknown, 3,6,4, and 7. The last five groups have sharply higher death rates with Risk 7 (moribund) giving 42.4% ...the death rates do not change much from one anesthetic group to another... In the low-risk code (1,2,5, unknown) patients, halothane, cyclopropane, and nitrous oxide have very similar rates for these high death operations.*

## Use of Contingency Tables

A contingency table is an important tool to present relationships between categories of information such as analgesic pain relief (yes/no) categorized by gender (male/female).[31] An N × N contingency table illustrates the relationship where N equals the number of categories. The display of the data is sometimes called a cross tabulation. Table 7-8 represents a cross tabulation of pain relief and gender using a 2 × 2 contingency table.

**Table 7-8** A 2 × 2 Contingency Table Showing the Relationship between Pain Relief and Gender[31]

|  | **Pain Relief** | | |
| --- | --- | --- | --- |
| **Gender** | **Yes** | **No** | **Totals** |
| Male | 88 (44%) | 112 (56%) | 200 (67%) |
| Female | 60 (60%) | 40 (40%) | 100 (33%) |
| Totals | 148 (49%) | 152 (51%) | 300 (100%) |

Contingency table analysis identifies possible differences in responses when patients are divided into subgroups. In Table 7-8, the contingency table shows if the response to the analgesic is different in males versus females. According to the table, a difference may exist because a higher percentage of females (60%) than males (44%) reported pain relief. This difference should be examined statistically with a significance test such as Chi square or Fisher's exact test to ensure that it is not a chance occurrence (*see* Chapter 8, Question 20).

A possible danger of contingency table analysis is the identification of subgroup differences that may not be important. An example is a phenomenon known as Simpson's paradox. In this phenomenon, differences noted when patients are divided into subgroups disappear when the subgroups are combined. Simpson's paradox occurs when there is a stronger relationship between the characteristics in the subgroup than in the group as a whole. With the data in Table 7-8, Simpson's paradox may occur if significantly more men were assigned to the experimental rather than the control group. Thus, the patients in the experimental group (who would be predominantly male) would be less responsive than the control group to the analgesic drugs used in the clinical drug trial.[31]

## Use of Figures and Graphs

A figure or graph presents a quick, easy-to-understand visual impression of the results. While such displays do not provide the detail found in tables or text, figures and graphs clarify or reinforce conclusions. In addition, graphical displays tend to be more effective than tables or text at drawing attention to important characteristics. Several helpful guidelines should be ollowed to ensure that figures and graphs are used properly (Table 7-9). Like tables, figures and graphs should be clear enough to be self-explanatory and not dependent on related information provided in the text.[6,9,10,17,18]

## Examples of Figures and Graphs

There are numerous ways to illustrate the data; the choice of what to use usually depends on the investigator's preference and purpose. Some common methods are histograms, scatter plots, line graphs, pie charts, and survival curves. The choice of which method to use is usually based on the type of data to be displayed.

### Histograms and bar graphs

Histograms and bar graphs are most effective in displaying information if the intervals are of equal width.[6,10,17,18] Figure 7-8 shows the hypothetical data set of 12 weekly diastolic blood pressure readings of one individual after initiation of new antihypertensive drug therapy. The histogram shows a slight trend toward a lower diastolic pressure.

Figure 7-8 shows the patient response with the maximum range of data points on the *y*-axis and *x*-axis. However, when the scale on the *y*-axis is reduced to cover only the range of the actual blood pressure readings, a different impression is given (Figure 7-9). The trend toward reduction in diastolic blood pressure appears to be more dramatic.

**Table 7-9** Guidelines for Proper Use of Figures and Graphs[6]

| Guideline | Description |
| --- | --- |
| Title | Clear and brief description of what the graphic display depicts. |
| Axes | Horizontal and vertical axes should be clearly defined and labeled. Zero points of both axes should be provided if appropriate. The units of measure on all scales, axes, rows, or columns should be easily visible and understandable. |
| Spacing of data | The number scales assigned to each axis should be appropriately spaced to cover the range of data collected. The scales should be of equal interval or space without exaggerating one part of the scale. Comparison of two different sets of data should be on the same scale. |
| Excluding data | "Broken" lines should be used to clearly indicate if a range of data or specific "data outliers" are not included in the axis. These breaks, usually shown by two slash marks, should be clearly noted. |
| Symbols | Symbols used in the graphic display need to be explained clearly. |
| Source of data | The source of the data should be clearly described, including the number of patients or observations that contributed to the display. |
| Differentiating data curves | An easily understood method of distinguishing data curves (such as different symbols) must be used when two or more curves are displayed. |
| Standard deviations | Should be included where appropriate to demonstrate the variability of the data. |

While the reduced scaling exaggerates the change in diastolic blood pressure from baseline, it is justifiable because of the narrow range of scores with no outliers. In addition, the scales are still evenly spaced. However, histograms with irregular or relatively small intervals on either the *x*- or *y*-axis would be inappropriate because the data may be distorted. Thus, the intervals chosen should reflect the data collected, and intervals containing small numbers and irregular scales should be avoided.

**Figure 7-8** Histogram of Patient Responses to Antihypertensive Drug (Normal Scale)

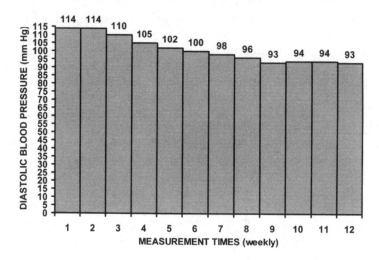

**Figure 7-9** Histogram of Patient Responses to Antihypertensive Drug (Adjusted Scale)

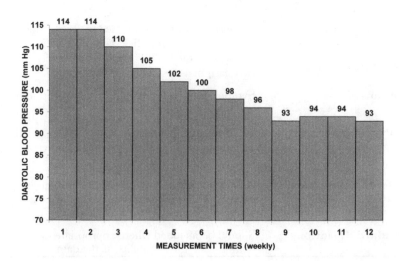

### Scatter diagrams and plots

Scatter diagrams and plots demonstrate the relationship between two measures relatively simply.[6,18,19] They are especially useful in displaying the relationship if there are relatively few data points. The example shown in Figure 7-10 illustrates a hypothetical relationship between a new lipid-lowering drug and serum triglycerides. The various triglyceride levels are plotted against the increasing drug dose. Although not always done, the  various data points are connected to better show the relationship. As indicated, the increasing doses of the drug were associated with a decreasing level of serum triglycerides. Unlike the histogram in Figure 7-9, the trend appears more realistic because the range of scores is large and larger intervals are used in the *y*-axis.

**Figure 7-10** Scatter Plot of Relationship between Serum Triglyceride Level and Increasing Drug Doses (N = 100)

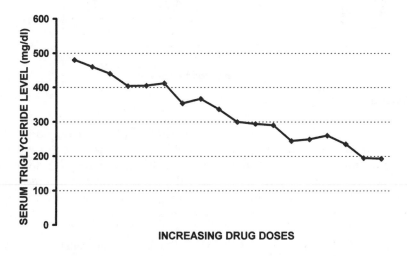

### Line graphs

Line graphs are similar to scatter plots and compare two types of data on the same graph (Figure 7-11).[17] Line graphs can be used for larger sets of data than scatter diagrams can. The line graph shown in Figure 7-11 compares the hypothetical effectiveness of an investigational drug with a control treatment for hypertension. The illustration includes a number of other features to make it more understandable. Each line is clearly marked to identify the responses due to the investigational drug and to the control drug. The number of patients in each group is shown in parentheses. The standard deviation (SD) of each mean score is reported to show the variability. The figure shows that the investigational drug appears to be more effective at reducing diastolic blood pressure than the control drug. In addition, the variability of the patients receiving the investigational drug appears to be greater than for the patients receiving the control drug. This finding suggests that the range of patient responses to the investigational drug compared to the control drug was greater.

**Figure 7-11**   Line Graph Comparing Patient Blood Pressure Responses to Investigational and Control Drug

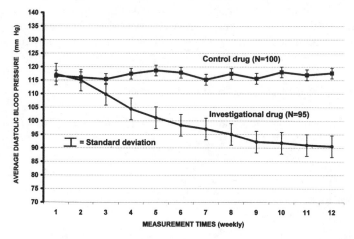

### Pie charts

Pie charts provide a useful method of displaying categorical data such as percentages of male/female, cure/no cure, and different types of ADEs (Figure 7-12).[14] Pie charts are most effective when providing an overview. Although easy to understand, the charts need to be constructed carefully. Use of a large number of categories can be confusing, and segments of similar size are difficult to distinguish.

**Figure 7-12**   Pie Chart Showing the Safety Profile of a New Antiarthritic Drug (N = 205)

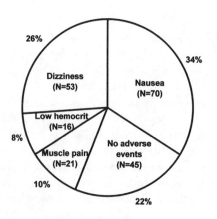

The pie chart in Figure 7-12 represents the proportion of patients who experienced various ADEs after taking an investigational drug. The chart clearly shows the distribution of patients. A number of other features are added to provide more information. The percentage of patients in each group is reported along with the actual number. The total sample of patients is reported in the title. The chart clearly indicates that most patients who received the drug experienced an ADE, with dizziness and nausea being the most common. In this example, there was no overlap in the categories based on the assumption that the patients experienced only one ADE, which rarely occurs in a clinical drug trial. Thus, the pie chart becomes more confusing when patients experience multiple ADEs.

### Survival curves

Survival curves estimate the likelihood of survival for a group of patients and are especially useful in studies of life-threatening illnesses such as AIDS or various forms of cancer.[14,21,22] A common type is the Kaplan-Meier estimated survival curve. As indicated in Figure 7-13, the curve is used to compare the likelihood of survival for a group of patients diagnosed with lymphoma and presenting clinical symptoms. The horizontal axis represents the time since diagnosis, while the vertical axis represents the probability of survival. According to the figure, 60% of patients suffering from clinical symptoms of lymphoma survive at least one year but less than 40% survive for three or more years following diagnosis.

**Figure 7-13** Sample Survival Curve for 31 Patients Diagnosed with Lymphoma and Presenting with Clinical Symptoms[a]

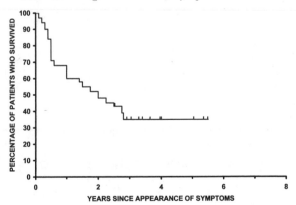

[a] Adapted with permission from Figure 6.1 in Matthews DE, Parwell VT. *Using and Understanding Medical Statistics.* 2nd ed. Basel, Switzerland: S. Karger AG. 1988: 68.

The data presented in the curve could be used graphically to assess the relative clinical efficacy of two drug treatments. An example is the clinical drug trial that compared two cancer chemotherapy combinations, cisplatin with cyclophosphamide and cisplatin with paclitaxel, for the treatment of ovarian cancer. The primary outcome measure was reduced mortality attributed to the ovarian cancer. The authors used the survival curve shown in Figure 7-14 as one means of showing the relative effects of the two combinations on four-year survival rates. As indicated, the survival rate for the group receiving the cisplatin–paclitaxel combination was higher than the survival rate for patients receiving the cyclophos-phamide–cisplatin combination, although the actual proportion of patients who died was about the same at four years.[32]

Although designed to assess mortality rates and patterns, the Kaplan-Meier curve is useful for analyses of clinical outcomes besides death. An example is the comparison of the effectiveness of felbamate to placebo in the treatment of partial seizures in patients undergoing presurgical evaluation. In this study, the survival curve shown in Figure 7-15 was used to analyze the length of time before the patient reached a maximum of four seizures. As indicated, patients in the placebo group experienced a fourth seizure more frequently and earlier than patients in the felbamate group.[33]

**Figure 7-14** Survival Curve for Comparing the Effectiveness of the Combination of Cisplatin and Cyclophosphamide with Cisplatin and Paclitaxel[a]

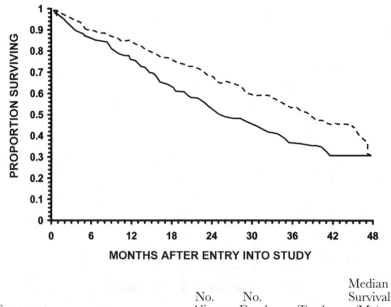

| Treatment | No. Alive | No. Dead | Total | Median Survival (Mo) |
|---|---|---|---|---|
| — Cisplatin + cyclophosphamide | 65 | 137 | 202 | 24 |
| - - Cisplatin + paclitaxel | 86 | 98 | 184 | 38 |

[a]Adapted with permission from Figure 2 in McGuire WP, Hoskins WJ, Brady MF, et al. Cyclophosphamide and cisplatin compared with paclitaxel and cisplatin in patients with stage III and stage IV ovarian cancer. *N Engl J Med*. 1996; 334:1–6.

**Figure 7-15** Survival Curve for Comparing the Effectiveness of Felbamate versus Placebo in Seizure Control[a]

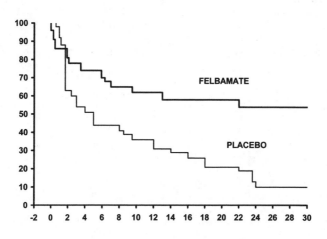

[a]Adapted with permission from Figure 1 in Bourgeois B, Leppik IE, Sackellares JC, et al. A double blind controlled trial in patients undergoing presurgical evaluation of partial seizures. *Neurology*. 1993; 43:693–6.

# References

1. Elenbaas RM, Elenbaas JK, Cuddy PG. Evaluating the medical literature, part II: statistical analysis. *Ann Emerg Med.* 1983; 12:610–20.

2. Bailar JC, Mosteller F. Guidelines for statistical reporting in articles for medical journals. In: Bailar JC, Mosteller F, eds. *Medical Use of Statistics*. Boston: NEJM Books; 1992:313–31.

3. O'Brien PC, Shampo MA. Statistics for clinicians: introduction. *Mayo Clin Proc.* 1981; 56:45–6.

4. Gaddis ML, Gaddis GM. Introduction to biostatistics: part 1, basic concepts. *Ann Emerg Med.* 1990; 19:86–9.

5. Berzon RA. Understanding and using health-related quality of life instruments within clinical research studies. In: Staquet MJ, Hays RD, Fayers PM, eds. *Quality of Life Assessment in Clinical Trials*. New York: Oxford University Press; 1998:3–15.

6. Bolton S. *Pharmaceutical Statistics*. 2nd ed. New York: Marcel Dekker; 1990.

7. Gehlbach SH. *Interpreting the Medical Literature: A Clinician's Guide: Practical Epidemiology for Clinicians*. 2nd ed. New York: Macmillan; 1988:70–4.

8. Riegelman RK, Hirsch RP. *Studying a Study and Testing a Test: How to Read the Medical Literature*. 2nd ed. Boston: Little Brown; 1989.

9. De Muth JE; *Basic Statistics and Pharmaceutical Statistical Applications*. New York: Marcel Dekker; 1999.

10. Pocock SJ. Basic principles of statistical analysis. In: Pocock SJ, ed. *Clinical Trials: A Practical Approach*. New York: Wiley, 1983:188–209.

11. Kramer MS, Shapiro SH. Scientific challenges in the application of randomized trials. *JAMA*. 1984; 252:2739–45.

12. Norman GR, Streiner DL. *PDQ Statistics*. Philadelphia: BC Decker; 1986.

13. Gaddis GM, Gaddis ML. Introduction to biostatistics: part 2, descriptive statistics. *Ann Emerg Med.* 1990; 19:309–15.

14. Matthews DE, Farwell VT. *Using and Understanding Medical Statistics*. 2nd ed. Switzerland: Karger; 1988.

15. O'Brien PC, Shampo MA. Statistics for clinicians: 1. Descriptive statistics. *Mayo Clin Proc*. 1981; 56:47–9.

16. Hays WL; *Statistics*. 4th ed. Orlando: Holt, Rinehart and Winston; 1993.

17. O'Brien PC, Shampo MA. Statistics for clinicians: 2. Graphic displays-histograms, frequency polygons, and cumulative distribution polygons. *Mayo Clin Proc*. 1981; 56:126–8.

18. O'Brien PC, Shampo MA. Statistics for clinicians: 3. Graphic displays-scatter diagrams. *Mayo Clin Proc*. 1981; 56:196–7.

19. Bennett RW, Popovich NG. Statistical inference as applied to bioavailability data—a guide for the practicing pharmacist. *Am J Hosp Pharm*. 1977; 34:712–23.

20. Moses LE. Statistical concepts fundamental to investigations. In: Bailar JC, Mosteller F, eds. *Medical Use of Statistics*. Boston: NEJM Books, 1992:5–25.

21. Campbell MJ, Machin D. *Medical Statistics: A Commonsense Approach*. New York: Wiley; 1990.

22. Morton RF, Hebel JR, McCarter RJ. *A Study Guide to Epidemiology and Biostatistics*. 4th ed. Gaithersburg MD: Aspen; 1996.

23. Peace KE. Design and analysis considerations for safety data, particularly adverse events. In: Solgliero-Gilbert G, ed. *Drug Safety Assessment in Clinical Trials*. 3rd ed. New York: Marcel Dekker; 1993:305–16.

24. Gaddis ML, Gaddis GM. Introduction to biostatistics: part 6, correlation and regression. *Ann Emerg Med*. 1990; 19:1462–3.

25. Liebetrau AM. *Measures of Association*. Newbury Park CA: Sage Publications; 1983.

26. O'Brien PC, Shampo MA. Statistics for clinicians: 7. regression. *Mayo Clin Proc*. 1981; 56:452–4.

27. Elwood MJ. *Critical Appraisal of Epidemiological Studies and Clinical Trials*. New York: Oxford University Press; 1998:3–13.

28. Hamilton CW. How to write and publish scientific papers: scribing information for pharmacists. *Am J Hosp Pharm*. 1992; 49:2477–84.

29. Mosteller F. Writing about numbers. In: Bailar JC, Mosteller F, eds. *Medical Use of Statistics*. Boston: NEJM Books; 1992: 375–89.

30. Ehrenberg ASC. The problem of numeracy. *Am Stat*. 1981; 35:67–71.

31. Zelterman D, Louis TA. Contingency tables in medical studies. In: Bailar JC, Mosteller F, eds. *Medical Use of Statistics*. Boston: NEJM Books; 1992: 293–311.

32. McGuire WP, Hoskins WJ, Brady MF, et al. Cyclophosphamide and cisplatin compared with paclitaxel and cisplatin and cisplatin in patients with stage III and stage IV ovarian cancer. *N Engl J Med*. 1996; 334:1–6.

33. Bourgeois B, Leppik IE, Sackellares JC, et al. A double blind controlled trial in patients undergoing presurgical evaluation of partial seizures. *Neurology*. 1993; 43:693–6.

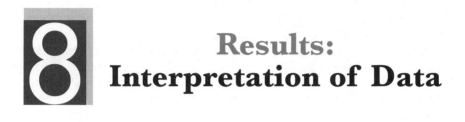

# 8 Results:
# Interpretation of Data

□

> □20. Are the statistical comparisons between the investigational drug and the control treatment appropriate?

> □21. Are the differences reported between the investigational drug and the control treatment statistically significant and interpreted correctly?

□

A clinical drug trial should determine whether an investigational drug is superior in efficacy and safety to existing treatments for a particular disorder. From a statistical standpoint, this approach involves the process of inference, in which conclusions are derived from imperfect or incomplete data.[1-4]

This chapter focuses on the investigator's approach to analyzing the differences between the investigational drug and the control treatment, especially on clinical efficacy and safety outcomes (Question 20). It addresses the statistical framework that is the basis of this approach and the various types of tests used to minimize a biased analysis. The remainder of the chapter addresses the issue of interpreting the results in an unbiased manner (Question 21). Concepts such as statistical and clinical significance are covered along with an examination of the effects of the sample size and the use of confidence intervals.

The clinical drug trial compares the effects of the investigational drug to the control treatment under similar research conditions. The methodology includes features to ensure that an unbiased comparison is made. Once the data are collected, organized, and summarized, the next step is the use of inferential statistics, also known as inductive statistics or tests of significance.[5-7]

These statistics are based on the science of drawing inferences under conditions of uncertainty, which means that conclusions about the possible differences between the investigational drug and control treatment are likely to be true if supported by unbiased use of proper statistical comparisons.

Good statistical methods offer the power to get the most information out of a given set of data through efficient design and evaluation. The term "inferential" implies that the validity of conclusions derived from the data is based on rules of probability. The use of these statistics enables various investigators to compare the effects of the investigational drug and control treatment in a consistent, although not completely standardized, manner. These tests minimize investigator bias. However, the proper use of inferential statistics is not a substitute for good experimental technique and does not replace sound professional judgment in the interpretation of trial results.[8,9]

The two fundamental issues that need to be addressed prior to the use of inferential statistics are methodological limitations in data collection and data management after collection. Data collected under poor research conditions such as unblinded observations, biased selection of subjects, or poorly managed data collection procedures will probably be poor and undoubtedly full of biases. Even if the trial methodology is appropriate, the investigator's approach to managing the data may be prone to distortions.[9]

The investigator's plan for the analysis, including the choice of statistical tests, should be initially described and justified in the methods section of an article. Explanations should be provided for any analyses described in the methods section that were not implemented or were only partially completed.[9]

## ☑ 20. Are the statistical comparisons between the investigational drug and the control treatment appropriate?

The statistical comparisons of the effects of the investigational and the control treatment are based on the scientific principle of hypothesis testing. The trial hypotheses, usually represented by the study objectives, provide the framework for the statistical comparison. Once that framework is established, the investigator chooses the approach to statistically compare the investigational and control groups. The approach includes the choice of the best statistical tests and the appropriate number of analyses to compare the responses of the experimental and control groups. This process is not standardized but depends on the nature of the data and the preferences of the investigator. Nevertheless, it should be relatively common because the Food and Drug Administration (FDA) discourages nontraditional approaches.[10]

Inferential statistics involves using tests designed to limit the possibility that the differences observed between the experimental and control groups are due to a chance occurrence and not because of the investigational drug. Statistical testing usually involves the establishment of a hypothesis that contains a quantitative statement about an effect. A hypothesis is assumed by the investigator to be true until otherwise proven differently. An example would be the hypothesis that a new antihypertensive drug would show a statistically significant decrease in diastolic blood pressure compared to the control treatment. Hypotheses are rarely stated in a clinical drug trial because they are based on relatively narrow statistical assumptions. Instead, hypotheses are represented by the study objectives. Trial objectives should be precisely written to represent the study hypotheses clearly.

The study objectives usually represent the research or alternate hypothesis (sometimes designated as $H_1$). However, the statistical tests examine the null or statistical hypothesis (sometimes designated as $H_o$) derived from the research hypothesis. In the antihypertensive drug example, the null hypothesis would be that there are no differences between the experimental group receiving the investigational drug and the control group receiving another treatment.[3,11,12]

The null hypothesis, as opposed to the research hypothesis, is tested statistically because it is mathematically less complex. Only one type of difference occurs with the null hypothesis (no difference), whereas a wide range of differences can occur with the research hypothesis. Nevertheless, the null hypothesis and the research hypothesis are roughly opposite. Thus, if the null hypothesis is "accepted," the research hypothesis must be "rejected." In contrast, the rejection of the null hypothesis does not necessarily mean that the research hypothesis is true because of the infinite range of possible alternate hypotheses besides those stated by the investigator.

The basic regulatory assumptions of investigational drugs tested in phase III and IV clinical trials are that the drug is considered safe but not efficacious until proven otherwise. Thus, the null hypotheses would be "the drug is safe" and "the drug is not efficacious." The alternate hypotheses, based on the regulatory assumptions, would be "the drug is not safe" and "the drug is efficacious," respectively. For a sponsor's drug to be approved as efficacious, enough information must be accumulated to contradict the null hypothesis. Rejection of the null hypothesis indicates that a significant difference exists between the experimental and control groups and that the difference is not due to chance alone.[10,13]

One important issue in developing hypotheses is whether they were developed before or after the research began. Hypotheses developed before the research began are *a priori* hypotheses, and hypotheses developed after the data are collected are *post hoc* or *post priori* hypotheses. It is wise to regard any conclusions based on *post hoc* hypotheses cautiously. These conclusions are more likely based on chance occurrence than those based on the original hypothesis. Unplanned statistical analyses or *post hoc* analyses are sometimes referred to as "data dredging" or "data snooping" and should be viewed as the basis for future confirmatory research rather than as facts. Investigators commonly do not distinguish between the two types of hypotheses. However, any deviation in the original research protocol must be approved by the FDA. Investigators should be candid in describing what part of their analysis was planned and what was not planned.[1,2,11,14–16]

Inferential statistics are designed to minimize falsely rejecting or accepting the null hypotheses. Two types of interpretive errors are possible. A Type I or alpha error occurs when the investigator concludes that an actual difference existed between the experimental and control groups when, in fact, it did not. This interpretation is also known as falsely rejecting the null hypothesis of no difference. A Type II or beta error occurs when the investigator concludes that no difference existed between the trial groups when, in fact, it did. This error is also known as falsely accepting the null hypothesis of no difference. Type I and II errors are directly related. An increase in Type I error probability decreases Type II error probability if other design factors are constant. The probability of making a Type I or alpha error is represented by the p value. Statistical significance is traditionally set at a p value of 0.05 (i.e., $p < 0.05$), which means that the investigator is 95% confident that a Type I error was not made.

Investigators need to establish how much error they are willing to accept before the initiation of the study. Investigators usually focus on statistical tests that examine the likelihood of a Type I error occurring and frequently do not assess the probability that a Type II error will occur. However, ignoring Type II errors would be a serious oversight because undetected, but "actual," differences may be important in practice or because further evaluation of a promising investigational drug may seem unwarranted.[2,10,11,17–21]

For assessment of drug efficacy in the drug approval process, a Type I error is synonymous with the FDA's incorrect interpretation of an investigational drug's efficacy (and subsequent marketing approval), and a Type II error is synonymous with the sponsor's risk of failing to detect a truly efficacious drug. For safety, a Type I error is synonymous with the sponsor's failing to show the drug is safe, while a Type II error is the FDA's decision to allow marketing of an unsafe drug.[10]

Investigators usually do not provide significant discussion about the probability of a Type I or II error occurring. Thus, the reader should consider the possibility while examining results. Type I errors should be considered whenever claims of superior efficacy and safety of the investigational drug are made, while Type II errors should be considered if the clinical trial results show no differences between the investigational drug and active control treatment.

## Choice of Statistical Tests

The choice of what statistical tests to use for comparing the investigational drug and control should be part of the clinical research plan and should be based on the study objectives, the study design, and the characteristics of the data collected. In some cases, the tests are modified because of changes in the study protocol (e.g., failure to reach patient enrollment goals or significant patient withdrawal) or based on preliminary data analysis.

Many tests determine whether the null hypothesis is true. The objective would be to select the most effective test for detecting true differences between the experimental and control groups. Investigators tend to avoid highly sophisticated statistical procedures unless they are widely accepted by the scientific community and the FDA. If possible, the statistical approach and the model underlying the analysis should be justified and documented by literature references. Multiple statistical approaches are often used so that the results achieved with one statistical method can be verified with another method. This approach allows the investigator to try both traditional and new, perhaps more sophisticated, techniques to examine the differences between the groups.[9]

The effect of using the wrong type of significance test depends partially on the magnitude of the difference between the experimental and control groups. The choice of tests is less important if the different tests give essentially the same result. The selection of the proper test is important, however, where there is a strong likelihood that different results will occur depending on the test used. Thus, investigators may choose to report or emphasize only those statistical tests that support their hypotheses.[2,22,23]

Ideally, investigators should refrain from simply stating what test of significance was used during the statistical analysis. Statements such as "we used t tests, chi-square, and Fisher's exact test" are acceptable only if supplemented with a clear description of the statistical analysis plan. Although often limited by journal space restrictions, investigators should discuss their assumptions about the data and the expectations regarding the direction in which the effect will occur.[24,25]

The investigator should consider various factors in the choice of the best statistical test (or tests) of significance to use, such as

- parametric versus nonparametric tests,
- tests used for single versus multiple comparisons,
- one-sided versus two-sided tests, and
- tests used for measuring relative risk.

The choice is usually based on the study objectives, trial methodology, type of data collected, and investigator's preferences.

### *Parametric versus nonparametric tests*

Based on the characteristics of the data collected, significance tests can be divided into parametric and nonparametric tests.[2,12,15,22,23,26,27]

Parametric tests require specific assumptions about the data collected. Nonparametric tests are recommended if the distribution of data is unknown or the data do not meet the criteria necessary for parametric tests. Parametric tests are more powerful than nonparametric tests in identifying "real" differences between the experimental and control groups.

While the differences between the two types of tests appear clear, sometimes the tests are applied incorrectly to the wrong type of data. The problem is more serious if a parametric test is used when a nonparametric test is more appropriate, because the potential violations of the test's assumptions may distort the results. Conversely, the use of a nonparametric test instead of the more appropriate parametric test may result in a less exact analysis of the differences between the study groups.[27]

### Parametric tests

The basic assumptions needed to use parametric tests are[2,5,7,13,15,17,21,22,28–30]

- data collected are normally distributed,
- variability of the data collected from the experimental and control groups is roughly equal,
- measures of patient response are independent and not related in any manner, and
- data are continuous with interval or ratio scales.

The tests are useful even if all these assumptions are not strictly met. The only assumption that cannot be violated is the use of independent measures. "Independence" means the results of one measure are not dependent on the results of the other. An example of a dependent measure would be comparing two measures of the same patient taken at separate times.[2,5,7,13,15,17,21,22,28–30]

The most commonly used parametric tests are the student t test and analysis of variance. The student t test (commonly referred to as the t test) is the suggested approach when the investigator is making a single comparison between the experimental and control groups. The paired t test is a modification used with dependent measures (e.g., comparison of baseline responses with responses after the drug is administered). The paired t test assumes that the mean for one set of data is closely related to the other set of data. An example would be measures of the same patient's blood pressure taken at the beginning and end of a clinical drug trial.[2,13,21,22]

The accepted method of analysis for comparing three or more groups is analysis of variance (ANOVA), which has advantages over multiple t tests (Table 8-1). Because it is exactly the same as the t test,

ANOVA is rarely used for the comparison of two groups. ANOVA compares the variability of the subjects within each group to each other and to subjects in the other trial groups. Like the t test, ANOVA is effective even if most assumptions for parametric tests are not strictly met, with the exception of the assumption of independent measures.[2,15,28–30]

**Table 8-1** Advantages of Analysis of Variance Compared to Multiple t Tests [2,15,28–30]

| Advantage | Description |
| --- | --- |
| Probability of Type I error | Reduced likelihood of making a Type I error as the number of comparisons increases |
| Calculation | Less cumbersome to calculate |
| Detection | More powerful in detecting group differences |
| Examining multiple independent effects | One type of ANOVA (two-way) analyzes different effects without increasing the chance of a Type I error occurring |

The ANOVA procedure determines the probability that nonchance differences occurred among treatment groups. The specific differences and the extent of these differences are determined by another set of related statistical tests. These tests, collectively called multiple comparison tests, are available in various forms such as the least significant difference (LSD), Duncan's multiple range test, Nueman-Keuls test, Tukey's multiple range test, Bonferroni t procedure, and the Scheffe' procedure. All comparison tests are based on the t test but include corrections for the multiple comparisons being made and the increased likelihood of identifying "false" differences. The tests vary in how conservative they are in detecting differences. The choice of test is generally based on the investigator's concern about the negative consequences of making either a Type I or II error.[2,5,15,17,29]

ANOVA statistical designs vary in complexity. The least complicated approach is one-way ANOVA, an expansion of the student t test to more than two groups. A typical one-way ANOVA design for a clinical drug trial compares three different drug treatments in different trial groups but at the equivalent dose schedule. A more complex approach would be the two-way ANOVA, in which the investigator is interested in examining the effects of drugs used in factorial designs (*see* Chapter 4, Question 10). Unlike the one-way version, which focuses on one level of each treatment (e.g., one dose level of each of three different drugs used), two-way ANOVA examines multiple levels (e.g., two dose levels as well as the three different drugs). The analysis determines the "main effects" of the model (e.g., relative effectiveness of each drug compared to each other) and "interaction effects" (e.g., whether the relative effectiveness is altered by increasing the dose of each drug).[7]

Another type of ANOVA, referred to as analysis of covariance (ANCOVA), adjusts for important baseline differences among the trial groups. ANCOVA removes the influence of these differences from the analysis of the reported results (*see* Chapter 4, Question 12). Other more complex ANOVA designs not typically used in clinical drug trials are hierarchical and split-plot factorial ANOVAs.[5,17,29,30]

### Nonparametric tests

Nonparametric tests[5–7,13,19,26,27] are useful when the characteristics of the data collected are not known or thought not to meet the assumptions required for use of parametric tests. The advantages of these tests are that they

- depend on a minimum number of data assumptions,

- can be quickly and easily performed,

- are easy to understand, and

- can be applied to measurements with a limited number of responses, such as nominally scaled data (for example, cure/no cure).

Their ease of application sometimes results in their use when parametric tests would be more appropriate. Nonparametric tests can also be tedious to compute mathematically.[7]

The most commonly used nonparametric tests are described in Table 8-2. As indicated, the tests vary by the type of data they analyze (e.g., nominal, ordinal, interval, or ratio), the number of groups compared (two or greater than two), and whether the data were collected from paired (same patient) or independent (different patient) samples. The most popular nonparametric test is the chi square, primarily because of its ease of use and comprehension.

### One-sided versus two-sided significance tests

Another criterion used for selection of the proper statistical test is whether the test should be one-sided (or tailed) or two-sided (or tailed).[2,5,13,28,31–36] Two-sided or two-tailed significance tests examine the probability that the investigational drug is superior or inferior to the control drug. A one-sided or one-tailed test assumes that a difference occurs in one direction, usually that the investigational drug is superior to the drug used in the control group.

One-sided tests are more powerful than two-sided tests because the focus on one direction reduces data variability. Despite the value of using a one-sided test, there are numerous limitations to its use (Table 8-3).

**Table 8-2** Nonparametric Tests

| Nonparametric Test | Description |
|---|---|
| **For two groups:** | |
| **Chi square** | Most common nonparametric test. Involves two discrete variables with nominal scales (or categories of continuous data separated into two parts). One variable is usually the study groups (experimental and control) and the other the clinical outcome (cure/no cure). Samples are independent. Analysis is performed most often with a $2 \times 2$ table. Need a minimum sample size of 20 (five in each cell). |
| **Fisher's exact** | Like the chi-square test, useful for comparing two discrete variables with nominal scales from independent measures. Very useful for sample sizes under 20. |
| **Kolmogorov-Smirnov** | Compares the differences between two study groups with respect to expected location and dispersion of data points. Data are compared with a theoretical distribution and must be at least ordinally scaled and from independent samples. |
| **McNemar's** | Examines for possible differences between related measures with nominal scales. The relationship is usually the same measure performed at baseline and after drug administration that contains nominal scales such as cure/no cure or absence/presence of symptom. |
| **Mann-Whitney U** | Tests for possible differences between groups from independent samples by ranking all scores and examining the relative ranks for each score. The variable measured is continuous with at least an ordinal scale. |
| **Wilcoxon matched-pairs signed rank** | Similar to Mann-Whitney test but applied to paired or related samples. Differences between group measures of continuous variables with interval scales are compared and ranked, including direction of distances. |
| **More than two groups:** | |
| **Friedman** | Applied to data that are ranked and organized. Like a two-way ANOVA with two factors being compared at two levels or with three or more groups. Useful when the parametric two-way ANOVA is not desirable. |
| **Kruskall-Wallis** | Extension of the Mann-Whitney U test to a comparison of more than two groups. |

**Table 8-3** Limitations of Using One-Sided Significance Tests

| Limitation | Description |
| --- | --- |
| Lack of uniformity | Arbitrary use of one-sided or two-sided tests creates an inconsistency in the reporting of p values. |
| Lack of theoretical support | Prior research or theory rarely enables the investigator to confidently predict that the investigational drug will only have a positive effect. |
| Exaggeration of differences | One-sided tests tend to exaggerate the importance of marginal differences. |

Two-sided tests are usually preferred in clinical drug trials because the expected possible outcomes may be in three (rather than one) separate directions: increase, decrease, or no change. Because of the potential for biased interpretations, the use of one-sided tests of significance should always be clearly noted by the investigator.[2,5,13,28,31–36]

## Choice of Risk Assessment Tests

Measures of risk are normally associated with epidemiological studies that examine disease patterns.[37–45] However, they are also used in clinical drug trials to assess the incidence of adverse drug events (ADEs), especially in phase IV or postmarketing surveillance studies. The statistics used are the relative risk and odds ratio. Although normally applied to comparisons of disease incidence when a specific factor is present or absent, the relative risk or risk ratio can be considered as the incidence (or prevalence) rate of ADEs among patients taking the investigational drug compared to the rate of ADEs in the control group. The odds ratio, an estimate of what happens when a patient begins taking the investigational drug, is similar to the relative risk ratio when the expected incidence is low.[37,38]

The relative risk is defined by

$$\text{relative risk} = \frac{\text{incidence of ADE in experimental group}}{\text{incidence of ADE in control group}}$$

An example would be a hypothetical situation where the prevalence of the ADE in the experimental group is 50% (odds 1:1) and in the control group is 25% (odds 1:3). The relative risk is 2 (prevalence of exposed/prevalence of unexposed = 50/25 = 2). No consistent guidelines indicate the appropriate size of the relative risk needed to suggest a causal relationship. Nevertheless, a relative risk ratio of 10 (meaning that the ADE is 10 times more likely to occur in the experimental group than in the control group) would be better than a relative risk ratio of 2. However, relative risk ratios are sometimes misleading in estimating the risk of experiencing an ADE because the actual prevalence is low. A relative risk ratio of 3 may appear to be important but may only indicate that the effect is likely to occur just three times in an experimental group of 1000 patients compared to once in a control group of similar size.[40-45]

The advantage of using the relative risk ratio is that an appropriate estimation of the risk associated with taking the investigational drug can be established, assuming other conditions are met. These conditions are that the patients in the trial are similar to the target population, that a consistent relationship is shown, and that a causal sequence is established[37] (*see* Chapter 9, Question 22).

The odds ratio estimates the relative risk of the ADE in patients who ultimately take the investigational drug in practice.[37] Two assumptions need to be fulfilled before the odds ratio is valid:

- The incidence of the ADE has to be relatively low.

- The control group should be representative of the target population.

The odds ratio is calculated by the following formula:

$$\text{odds ratio} = \frac{\text{experimental patients with ADE} \times \text{patients in control group without ADE}}{\text{experimental patients without ADE} \times \text{patients in control group with ADE}}$$

An example would be the previous hypothetical situation where the prevalence of the ADE in the experimental group is 50% (odds 1:1) and in the control group is 25% (odds 1:3). While the relative risk is 2, the odds ratio is 3 ($50 \times 75/25 \times 50 = 3750/1250 = 3$).

The odds ratio is a good estimate of relative risk in most situations, the exception being where the outcome is very frequent. However, in most situations the difference is small. Thus, the odds ratio is the statistic most reported.[37,38]

## Multiple Comparisons

The principal comparison in most clinical drug trials is the statistical examination of the differences between patient responses to the investigational drug and other patients' responses on the primary outcome measure. However, most clinical drug trials are costly and complex and to limit the analysis to one comparison would be inefficient. Thus, most clinical drug trials often include multiple comparisons of differences between the experimental and control groups.[16,46]

The value of multiple examinations of possible differences between the experimental and control groups is that clinical efficacy and safety of the investigational drug can be better defined. However, a significant limitation is the increased possibility of identifying false differences in the effects between the investigational drug and the control treatment (Type I error).[16,46]

Multiple examinations occur for various purposes. Many clinical trials have multiple objectives to analyze. One objective is usually designated as primary, and the others are designated as secondary. The potential for Type I error increases with the increase in the number of objectives. The other potential for Type I error occurs when no difference is reported in the primary outcome measure but is reported in at least one secondary objective.[16,47–49]

Another source for Type I error is the comparison of effects of more than two study groups. For example, a clinical drug trial could include three groups: patients receiving the investigational drug, patients receiving an active control drug, and patients receiving a placebo. Comparing just two groups simultaneously (using the student t or chi-square tests) increases the number of comparisons and the probability of a Type I error. Thus, the comparison should be made with statistical tests, such as analysis of variance or the Friedman test, designed to adjust for multiple simultaneous comparison of three or more study groups.

A major source of Type I error is subgroup analysis. Patients are divided into subgroups of patients (e.g., women, aged patients, patients with certain symptoms of the disease state, racial minorities) to determine whether they respond differently. The principal aim of subgroup analyses is to decide if there is a subset of patients for whom the investigational drug is clinically more efficacious or safer. While useful as a tool to understand the investigational drug's clinical effects, information from these subgroup results must be interpreted cautiously.[46]

Several critical issues need to be addressed in assessing the value of subgroup analyses. The first is whether the analyses was "planned" or not. Planned statistical analysis involves the development of hypotheses or objectives before the research and implementation of a structured analysis plan to test the hypotheses efficiently. Unplanned statistical analysis is less structured and more likely to identify chance differences between the experimental and control groups. It is important to avoid the situation in which the choice of subgroups is data driven; that is, when the types of subgroups appear to be selected based on observed statistical differences rather than on any preconceived hypotheses. This approach is often called data dredging or data snooping and is prone to significant biases.[1,2,11,14,16,28,46,50–52]

Few investigators reveal whether their subgroup analysis is planned or unplanned. However, some trial characteristics help the reader identify the type of subgroup analysis performed. They include the type of subgroups chosen, the use of stratified randomization to ensure the presence of key characteristics during the trial, sample size calculations performed before the trial to ensure a sufficient number of patients in each subgroup, and analyses performed to identify relatively infrequent events, such as a rare and unpredictable ADE.[1,2,11,14,16,28,46,50–52]

Regardless of whether the analysis is planned or not, there needs to be a biological or theoretical rationale for the choice of which subgroups to analyze. This rationale should be documented with references from previous research. Subgroups based on the amount of data collected, such as analysis of only those patients who completed the clinical drug trial, could result in biased interpretation because those patients could be substantially different from the patients who withdrew from the study[16,46](*see* Intention-to-Treat Analysis in Chapter 6, Question 17).

Finally, differences noted from subgroup analysis need to be compared with the potential differences noted on the primary outcome measures. A significant subgroup effect in the presence of an overall effect may be used to refine the primary hypotheses, while a subgroup difference noted in the absence of a significant overall effect is more difficult to detect and is more likely to be a chance occurrence.[16,46]

The large number of possible subgroups analyzed creates an opportunity to identify only those subgroups most responsive to the investigational drug, especially if the analysis is unplanned. These conclusions may be misleading. A tendency exists to concentrate on those responses most favorable to the investigator's hypotheses, even if the particular result has a low theoretical plausibility or lacks prior data to support it.[1,2,11,14,28,50–53]

## ☑ 21. Are the differences reported between the investigational drug and the control treatment statistically significant and interpreted correctly?

Once the appropriate statistical tests have been applied to the data, the investigator must interpret the results. While guidelines are available, most interpretation is subjective and based on various factors.[54–56] These factors include the statistical probability that true differences occurred, the quality of the study methodology used to collect the data, the worthiness of the data collection procedures, the size of the difference, and the clinical value of the results. The arbitrariness of this interpretation makes it prone to biases, quite often due to a lack of understanding about the statistical assumptions underlying the statistical tests.

### Statistical Significance

A statistically significant result means that there is a strong probability that the observed differences between the experimental and control groups are not due to chance. The probability is expressed by the p value that represents the likelihood of making a Type I error. The p value is widely misunderstood and interpreted several ways. To improve understanding, an attempt has been made to standardize certain interpretations (Table 8-4). According to these guidelines, statistical significance occurs with any p value less than 0.05, which generally means that the investigator is 95% confident that the differences observed are not due to chance. The choice of p <0.05 as statistically significant is an arbitrary cutoff originally developed in quality control studies where the emphasis was on making decisions for improving manufacturing. Thus, a p value such as p <0.055 is not considered statistically significant because it can be rounded to p <0.06, while p <0.054 is considered statistically significant because it can be rounded to p <0.05.[2,5,11,13,14,17,21,22,25,57,58]

**Table 8-4** Standard Interpretation of p Values[11,13]

| p Value | Interpretation |
| --- | --- |
| p = 0.06 and greater | Not statistically significant |
| 0.05> p >0.01 | Statistically significant[a] |
| 0.01> p >0.001 | Very statistically significant[b] |
| p <0.001 | Highly statistically significant[b] |

[a] The value is more commonly stated as p < 0.05. Thus, any value of p equal to 0.05 or less is considered statistically significant.
[b] The two interpretations are sometimes combined so that any value of p equal to 0.01 or less is considered highly statistically significant.

Despite attempts to standardize interpretation of p values, these values are often misinterpreted in clinical trial reports. Investigators sometimes place undue importance on a p value of 0.05 or less by implying that such a result, based on statistical significance alone, is clinically important. Statistical significance does not provide much information about the magnitude or importance of the observed difference. Rather, statistical significance indicates that a strong probability exists that a nonchance difference between the experimental and control groups was observed. The proper interpretation of statistically nonsignificant results is that a strong likelihood exists that no differences were observed between the experimental and controls groups. Investigators should refrain from merely stating that a result is "statistically significant" without stating the test statistic used and the observed p value. In addition, misleading statements such as "almost significant" or "there is a trend toward significance" for p values greater than 0.05 should be avoided. For studies in which no differences were found, discussion of the probability of making a Type II or beta error should be included.[2,11,13,14,25,57,58]

The p values are based on mathematical models or probability estimations and are the same for each significance test. The correctness of those values depends on the extent to which the underlying assumptions are met by the data collected. For parametric tests such as the t test or analysis of variance, these assumptions include normally distributed and continuously scaled data, independent measures, and equal variability among the trial groups. Significance tests do not address possible problems with the trial design, especially those problems that may result when study groups are not directly comparable. Any assessment of significance tests should review the steps the investigators took to ensure group comparability. Such steps include random assignment of patients, proper management of data collection, maintenance of similar patient dropout rates in each group, and analysis of possible group differences. Causal relationships are difficult to establish solely through the use of statistical tests [5,13,17,21,22,25] (*see* Chapter 9, Question 22).

## Effect of Sample Size

Statistical interpretation of the differences between the experimental and control groups is strongly influenced by the number of patients enrolled. An assessment of that influence can be made through the estimation of the power of a statistical test. Power is defined as the probability that the statistical test will detect true differences between the experimental and control groups (Type II or beta error) and is calculated by subtracting the Type II error probability from 1.[2,12,59-63]

The power of a statistical test depends on

- the size of the sample,

- the desired size of the difference to be detected,

- the amount of variation in the data collected, and

- the desired alpha level for making a Type I error (Table 8-5).

Several formulas are available to calculate the power of a statistical test, and the calculations are usually done before the trial begins. However, power calculations may also be done after the trial data have been collected, when more precise information needed for the calculation is usually available.[2,12,59-63]

**Table 8-5** Factors Influencing the Power of a Statistical Test

| Factor | Influence on Power |
|---|---|
| Sample size | Increases with the sample size |
| Size of difference | Increases as the expected size of the difference to be detected between the experimental and control groups increases |
| Variability | Increases as the variability among the data decreases |
| Type I (alpha) error | Increases as the probability of making a Type I error increases |

Unlike Type I or alpha errors, there is no traditional consensus about the acceptable level of power of a statistical test. The Type II error rate is often set at a maximum value of 20%, which sets the minimum acceptable power level at 80% (power = 1 − Type II error rate). The acceptance of setting the power level at 80% illustrates the greater emphasis that investigators put on avoiding Type I errors (with an acceptable level of 5%) than Type II errors. Reliance on a less conservative power level may result in investigators missing clinically important differences between the experimental and control groups or clinically important but relatively rare side effects.[17,19,62,64,65]

The primary way in which investigators avoid the effects of low statistical power is to enroll an adequate number of patients. Although the actual number enrolled is often influenced more by patient availability, cost constraints, trial duration, or government regulations, estimation of the desired number should be based on statistical theory. The statistical estimation is based on the variability of the data collected and the anticipated size of the differences to be detected.[17,19,62,64,65]

A hypothetical example of a sample size requirement for clinical efficacy is shown in Table 8-6. In the example, the effectiveness of a new antiarrhythmic drug in reducing the incidence of atrial fibrillation is compared to standard treatment. In this example, the incidence of atrial

**Table 8-6** Estimated Number of Patients Needed for the Control and Experimental Groups in a Hypothetical Clinical Trial of a New Antiarrhythmic Drug

| Incidence of AF[a] | | | Number of Patients Needed in Each Group[b] | | |
|---|---|---|---|---|---|
| EXP | CTL | DIFF | $N_{10}$[c] | $N_{20}$[d] | $N_{50}$[e] |
| 5 | 50 | 45 | 23 | 19 | 12 |
| 10 | 50 | 40 | 30 | 24 | 15 |
| 20 | 50 | 30 | 58 | 45 | 26 |
| 30 | 50 | 20 | 134 | 103 | 56 |
| 40 | 50 | 10 | 538 | 407 | 210 |
| 45 | 50 | 5 | 2130 | 1600 | 806 |

[a] Represents the percentage of patients in the sample with atrial fibrillation (AF). The percentage was held constant at 50% for patients in the control group (CTL) ; EXP = experimental group and DIFF = expected percentage difference between experimental and control groups.

[b] The number of patients needed is calculated from the formulas recommended by Borenstein and Cohen.[66] The chi-square statistic (with the Yates correction) is used to assess statistical significance. Power = 1 − beta (probability of Type II error). The p value is assumed to be equal to 0.05.

[c] $N_{10}$ is the power level of 0.90 and represents a 10% probability that a Type II error could occur.

[d] $N_{20}$ is the power level of 0.80 and represents a 20% probability that a Type II error could occur. It is the most commonly used level.

[e] $N_{50}$ is the power level of 0.50 and represents a 50% probability that a Type II error could occur.

fibrillation remains constant at 50% for the control group. The table indicates that a larger number of patients is needed as the expected difference between the experimental and control groups becomes smaller. In addition, increasing the power of the test requires increasing the number of patients enrolled.

Sample size is even more of a concern for identifying ADEs, especially the rare and unpredictable types. Although most investigators view power levels of 80% as satisfactory to determine whether the investigational drug is more clinically efficacious than the control treatment, the need to assess differences in drug safety between the study drugs may require a more sensitive test, especially for the relatively rare ADEs.[10]

As indicated in Table 8-7, the number of patients needed to receive the investigational drug to experience a rare (occurring in 0.1% of the patients) ADE is anywhere from approximately 2300 to 4600, depending on the degree of confidence (i.e., power level) desired. Detecting relatively infrequent ADEs (occurring in 1% of the patients) would require from 230 to 460 patients. Comparing the safety of the investigational drug to the control drug would require double the number indicated in the table to ensure adequate numbers of patients in the study group.

The information provided in Tables 8-6 and 8-7 supports the fact that most phase III and IV clinical drug trials are designed to assess clinical efficacy. A study designed to detect a 20% difference in clinical efficacy and at the expected 80% power level would include 103 patients per group. This number would be insufficient to detect ADEs that occur in 1% or less of the patients with any degree of confidence. Even larger clinical drug trials (300 patients in each study group) would only detect a small number of ADEs at the 99% level of confidence.

**Table 8-7** Estimated Number of Patients Needed to Identify the Percentage of Patients Who Will Experience a Specific ADE[10]

| Patients Who Will Experience an ADE | Patients Needed for Detection | | |
|---|---|---|---|
| | 90% Power Level | 95% Power Level | 99% Power Level |
| 0.1% | 2302 | 2995 | 4604 |
| 1% | 230 | 300 | 460 |
| 5% | 45 | 59 | 90 |
| 10% | 22 | 29 | 44 |
| 20% | 11 | 15 | 22 |
| 50% | 4 | 6 | 8 |

An example of a study designed to assess the incidence of ADEs is a clinical drug trial examining the effectiveness of multivitamin supplements in preventing neural tube defects in pregnant women. The clinical outcome measure was the incidence of neural tube defects, which had a prevalence rate of 5.7 per 1000 patients (0.57%) based on previous records.

Eventually, 4753 patients were enrolled and assigned relatively evenly to the experimental and control groups (2394 and 2310 patients, respectively). Based on the power analysis shown in Table 8-7, there should be enough patients to identity at least some neural tube defects. In fact, the experimental group experienced no neural tube defects and the control group experienced six (0.26%). Although the occurrence of the event was very rare, these results were statistically significant using the Fisher's exact test (p = 0.029).[67]

Investigators should describe how they addressed sample size issues and include that discussion in the methods section. This discussion should indicate whether the sample size calculations are based on the initial sample of patients needed for the trial or on the final sample who completed the study. Sometimes an additional 10 or 20% is added to the initial power calculations to ensure an adequate sample size by the time the study is completed. Even if this overestimation is present, the number of patients who completed the study should approximately equal the investigators' initial sample size calculations presented in the methods section.[10,70]

While a discussion of sample size is often omitted, the reader can still assess whether the number is adequate based on other information. In those studies in which there are no differences reported between the experimental and controls on the primary clinical outcome measures, the adequacy of the sample size should be addressed. This issue is particularly important if the investigational drug is compared to an active control. Even if differences are observed with groups consisting of small sample size, the effects may be overestimated due to the influence of outliers on the distribution of scores (*see* Chapter 7, Question 18)

An example of a statement of a power analysis was included in an article[68] describing the clinical effectiveness of sumatriptan for the treatment of headache:

> *Data on 280 patients were required to detect a 15 percent difference in the rate of relief of headache between the combination of 6 mg of sumatriptan and placebo and two 6-mg injections of sumatriptan with 80 percent power, at the two-sided 5 percent significance level. After allowances were made for comparison with placebo and 8 mg of sumatriptan and for patients who died, data on a total of 630 patients were required.*

The statement provides a great deal of information about the sample size estimations. The investigators noted that the minimum desired observed difference between the experimental and control groups was 15%. They also indicated that the estimation was based on a 5% probability (two-sided test) of making a Type I error and a 20% probability of making a Type II error. This calculation resulted in a desired sample size of 280 patients per sample group (sumatriptan versus placebo) in which an additional 13% was added to adjust for patient withdrawals. In reality, the patient enrollment and assignment were different. Three groups were used initially to receive one injection (sumatriptan 6 mg, sumatriptan 8 mg, and placebo) and were assigned according to blocked randomization, 423, 110, and 106 patients. The larger number of patients in the sumatriptan 6-mg group was intended to have sufficient sample size to assess the effects of a second dose of the drug. Thus, although comprehensive, the power analysis statement was somewhat misleading.

Clinical drug trials with low power are likely to report no differences between the experimental and control groups, even when actual differences exist. These results could impede future research on the investigational drug or misrepresent the actual differences between the drug and standard drug treatment. It is also possible that a large number of clinical drug trials could report conflicting results primarily because of the different number of subjects used in each trial.[28,58,62,69-71]

## Clinical Significance

Statistical significance represents a readily determinable value obtained using an appropriate mathematical model. However, the finding of a statistically significant difference between the experimental and control groups on the primary clinical outcomes measured only means that there is a low probability that the variation is a chance occurrence. This statistical calculation is sometimes used to imply that the results are clinically important. Such use of statistical significance is misleading and inappropriate. While assessment of clinical significance is based on the assumption that the results are statistically significant, statistically significant results are not always clinically important.

Clinical significance[4,9,12,13,20,27,29,45,58,68,71-79] represents the increased margin of clinical efficacy (or safety) produced by the investigational drug (when compared with placebo or a reference compound) considered sufficiently important to be recognized as a therapeutic advantage by experts on the disease. Such a standard should be developed prior to the start of the trial to avoid too small or too large a sample size and to increase the likelihood that statistically significant results will also be clinically relevant.

Statistical significance is determined quantitatively using precise guidelines. Clinical significance is more subjective and depends on the opinion of healthcare practitioners and patients. While judgment of statistical significance is based on a probability assessment of the results reported, clinical significance is based on previous reports (Table 8-8)

Results that are statistically important but are not supported by previous reports should be interpreted cautiously. Statistically significant differences are sometimes erroneously accepted as clinically important despite the presence of severe limitations in the trial methodology or in the analysis of the results.[12,20,29,41,73,74] Certain terms used by the investigator may be misleading. In particular, the word "significant" should be used carefully.[27]

**Table 8-8** Comparison of Statistical and Clinical Significance[74]

| Characteristic | Statistical Significance | Clinical Significance |
|---|---|---|
| Purpose | Detect nonchance differences | Assess importance of difference |
| Criteria | p <0.05 | Expert/personal opinion |
| Determinants | Sample size<br>Patient variability<br>Accurate/reliable measures | Extent of change in clinical practice or change in quality of life measures (e.g., improved patient comfort, mortality) |

The most exact use of the term concerns the differences noted from the patient sample selected for the study. Thus, it would be appropriate to report statistically significant results by stating that "there is a significant difference between the experimental and control groups on clinical efficacy." Use of the word "significance" elsewhere may be misleading unless it is part of the term "statistical significance" or "clinical significance."[27]

An important determinant of clinical significance is the magnitude of the difference observed between the experimental and control groups once statistical significance has been established (Table 8-8). Although this amount can be estimated quantitatively by using percentage differences or qualitatively by using past research experience, both methods are subjective and prone to significant bias. A more appropriate method would be the use of confidence intervals (CIs), which have an advantage compared to significance tests because they provide a range in which the actual difference is likely to exist. Like significance tests, the degree of confidence that the actual value is within the reported range of values is traditionally set at 95%.

A hypothetical example would be a clinical drug trial in which an investigational antihypertensive drug reduced diastolic blood pressure by 20% compared to control treatment. Because of sufficient sample size, the results were statistically significant ($p < 0.05$). The results would be more informative, however, if the confidence interval of the difference was also reported. In this case, the hypothetical confidence interval has a lower limit of change of 3% and an upper limit of 40%, with a 95% degree of confidence. Thus, there is a 95% chance that the difference between the groups is between 3% and 40%. The CI indicates that the difference may be clinically important, but the lower limit suggests that it may also be unimportant. Confidence intervals that include a 1 (such as a reported difference between 0.7% and 30%) suggest that the experimental and control groups are not different.

Another way to express the confidence interval is to compare the CIs of both the experimental and control groups. Using a hypothetical example with the same data as the previous one, the investigational antihypertensive drug reduced blood pressure by 25% (95% CI, 13–50%) and the control drug treatment by 5% (95% CI, 0–10%). Since the CIs do not overlap, the groups are considered different. However, the lower limit of the blood pressure decrease due to the investigational drug is very close to the upper limit of decrease for the control treatment, indicating that the group difference may be relatively small.

The past misuse of significance tests has generated numerous recommendations that the tests be replaced by confidence intervals, particularly in case-control or cohort studies. Although overdependence on significance tests leads to incomplete information, p values provide details typically not present when only confidence intervals are reported. The statement that p = 0.0001 gives a clear indication of the likelihood that the observed difference is not due to chance. In addition, significance tests are based on prespecified criteria that require clear-cut and explicit decisions about the data collected. Thus, it may be preferable to cite both significance tests and confidence intervals when reporting the results of the clinical drug trial.[12,13,45,58,75–79]

Effective use of both the p value and the confidence interval was demonstrated in the reported results of a clinical drug trial evaluating the effectiveness and safety of sumatriptan for the treatment of migraine headache.[68]

*As compared with the placebo group at 60 minutes (after treatment), 47% more patients (95% confidence interval, 38% to 57%) who had received 6 mg of sumatriptan and 54% more patients (95% confidence interval, 43% to 65%) who had received 8 mg of sumatriptan had improvements in the severity of headache (p<0.001 for both comparisons). A complete resolution of pain also occurred in a significantly higher proportion of patients treated with either dose of sumatriptan than of patients given placebo (p<0.001).*

# References

1. Bailar JC. Science, statistics, and deception. *Ann Intern Med.* 1986; 104:259–60.

2. Elenbaas RM, Elenbaas JK, Cuddy PG. Evaluating the medical literature, part II: statistical analysis. *Ann Emerg Med.* 1983; 12:610–20.

3. O'Brien PC, Shampo MA. Statistics for clinicians: introduction. *Mayo Clin Proc.* 1981; 56:45–6.

4. Feinstein AR. Clinical biostatistics IV: statistical "malpractice"—and the responsibility of a consultant. *Clin Pharmacol Ther.* 1970; 11:898–914.

5. Bolton S. *Pharmaceutical Statistics.* 2nd ed. New York: Marcel Dekker; 1990.

6. Hays WL; *Statistics.* 4th ed. Orlando: Holt, Rinehart and Winston; 1993.

7. De Muth JE. *Basic Statistics and Pharmaceutical Statistical Applications.* New York: Marcel Dekker; 1999.

8. DeMets D. Distinction between fraud, bias, errors, misunderstanding, and incompetence. *Controlled Clin Trials.* 1997; 18:637–50.

9. Kassalow LM. Statistical and data management: collaboration in clinical research. In: Gaurino RA, ed. *New Drug Approval Process: The Global Challenge*. 3rd ed. New York: Marcel Dekker; 2000:289–310.

10. Peace KE. Design and analysis considerations for safety data, particularly adverse events. In: Solgliero-Gilbert G, ed. *Drug Safety Assessment in Clinical Trials*. 3rd ed. New York: Marcel Dekker; 1993:305–316.

11. Bennett RW, Popovich NG. Statistical inference as applied to bioavailability data—a guide for the practicing pharmacist. *Am J Hosp Pharm*. 1977; 34:712–23.

12. Gaddis GM, Gaddis ML. Introduction to biostatistics: part 3, sensitivity, specificity, predictive value and hypothesis testing. *Ann Emerg Med*. 1990; 19:591–7.

13. Ware JH, Mosteller F, Delgaudo F, et al. P Values. In: Bailar JC, Mosteller F, eds. *Medical Use of Statistics*. Boston: NEJM Books; 1992:181–200.

14. Barnes RW. Understanding investigative clinical trials. *J Vasc Surg*. 1989; 9:609–18.

15. Gaddis GM, Gaddis ML. Introduction to biostatistics: part 4, statistical inference techniques in hypothesis testing. *Ann Emerg Med*. 1990; 19:820–5.

16. Zipfel A, Grob P. How much detail on confirmatory statistics and exploratory statistics must a statistical report contain? *Drug Info J*. 1995; 29:479–82.

17. Kirk RE. *Experimental Design*. 2nd ed. Pacific Grove CA: Brooks/Cole; 1982.

18. Gaddis GM, Gaddis ML. Introduction to biostatistics: part 2, descriptive statistics. *Ann Emerg Med*. 1990; 19:309–15.

19. Campbell MJ, Machin D. *Medical Statistics: A Commonsense Approach*. New York: Wiley; 1990.

20. O'Brien PC, Shampo MA. Statistics for clinicians: 8. Comparing two proportions: the relative deviate test and chi square equivalent. *Mayo Clin Proc*. 1981; 56:513–5.

21. O'Brien PC, Shampo MA. Statistics for clinicians: 5. One sample of paired observations (paired t test). *Mayo Clin Proc*. 1981; 56:324–6.

22. Boyce EG, Nappi JM. Is there significance beyond the t-test? *Drug Intell Clin Pharm*. 1988; 22:334–5.

23. Pathek D. Parametric vs nonparametric statistics: a dilemma for the clinical researcher. *Drug Intell Clin Pharm*. 1979; 13:441–2.

24. Moses LE. Statistical concepts fundamental to investigations. In: Bailar JC, Mosteller F, eds. *Medical Use of Statistics*. Boston: NEJM Books; 1992:5–25.

25. Henzel RE. *Tests of Significance*. Newbury Park CA: Sage Publications; 1976.

26. Gaddis GM, Gaddis ML. Introduction to biostatistics: part 5, statistical inference techniques in hypothesis testing with nonparametric data. *Ann Emerg Med*. 1990; 19:1054–9.

27. Daniel W. *Applied Nonparametric Statistics*. 2nd ed. Boston: PWS-Kent Publishing; 1990.

28. Pocock SJ. Current issues in the design and interpretation of clinical trials. *Br Med J*. 1985; 290:39–42.

29. Godfrey K. Comparing the means of several groups. *N Engl J Med*. 1985; 313:1450–6

30. Iverson GR, Norpoth H. *Analysis of Variance*. Newbury Park CA: Sage Publications; 1987.

31. Salsburg D. Use of restricted significance tests in clinical trials: beyond the one vs two-tailed controversy. *Controlled Clin Trials*. 1989; 10:71–82.

32. Boissel JP. Some thoughts on two-tailed tests (and two-sided designs). *Controlled Clin Trials*. 1988; 9:385–6.

33. Peace KE. Some thoughts on one-tailed tests. *Controlled Clin Trials*. 1988; 9:383–4.

34. Fleiss JL. One-tailed versus two-tailed tests: rebuttal. *Controlled Clin Trials*. 1988; 10:227–30.

35. Goodman S. One-sided or two-sided p values? *Controlled Clin Trials*. 1988; 9:387–8.

36. Mckinney WP, Young MJ, Hartz A, et al. The inexact use of Fisher's exact test in six major medical journals. *JAMA*. 1989; 261:3430–3.

37. Elwood MJ. *Critical Appraisal of Epidemiological Studies and Clinical Trials*. New York: Oxford University Press; 1998:37–54.

38. Morton RF, Hebel JR, McCarter RJ. *A Study Guide to Epidemiology and Biostatistics*. 4th ed. Gaithersburg MD: Aspen; 1996.

39. Hartzema AG, Porta MS, Tilson HH. *Pharmacoepidemiology: An Introduction.* 2nd ed. Cincinnati: Harvey Whitney Books; 1991.

40. Kramer MS, Shapiro SH. Scientific challenges in the application of randomized trials. *JAMA.* 1984; 252:2739–45.

41. Freedman LS. The effect of partial non-compliance on the power of a clinical trial. *Controlled Clin Trials.* 1990; 11:157–68.

42. Polk RE, Hepler CD. Controversies in antimicrobial therapy: critical analysis of clinical trials. *Am J Hosp Pharm.* 1986; 43:630–40.

43. Pocock SJ. *Clinical Trials: A Practical Approach.* New York: Wiley; 1983:111.

44. Hallstrom A, Davis K. Imbalance in treatment assignments in stratified blocked randomization. *Controlled Clin Trials.* 1988; 9:375–82.

45. Bailar JC, Mosteller F. Guidelines for statistical reporting in articles for medical journals. In: Bailar JC, Mosteller F, eds. *Medical Use of Statistics.* Boston: NEJM Books; 1992:313–31.

46. Scott PE, Campbell G. Interpretation of subgroup analyses in medical device clinical trials. *Drug Info J.* 1998; 32:213–20.

47. Davis CE. Secondary endpoints can be validly analyzed, even if the primary endpoint does not provide clear statistical significance. *Controlled Clin Trials.* 1997; 18:557–60.

48. O'Neill RT. Secondary endpoints cannot be validly analyzed if the primary endpoint does not demonstrate clear statistical significance. *Controlled Clin Trials.* 1997; 18:550–6.

49. Pocock SJ. Clinical trials with multiple outcomes: a statistical perspective on their design, analysis, and interpretation. *Controlled Clin Trials.* 1997; 18:530–45.

50. Saville DJ. Multiple comparison procedures: the practical solution. *Am Stat.* 1990; 44:174–80.

51. Thompson DW. Statistical criteria in the interpretation of epidemiologic data. *Am J Pub Health.* 1987; 77:191–4.

52. Tukey JW. Some thoughts on clinical trials, especially problems of multiplicity. *Science.* 1977; 198:679–84.

53. Oxman AD, Guyatt GH. A consumer's guide to subgroup analysis. *Ann Intern Med.* 1992; 116:76–84.

54. Gunn I.P. Evidence based practice, research, peer review, and publication. *Crna.* 1998; 9(4):177–82.

55. Pearson KC. Role of evidence-based medicine and clinical practice guidelines in treatment decisions. *Clin Ther.* 1998; 20:C80–C85.

56. Rosenberg WM, Sackett DL. On the need for evidence-based medicine. *Therapie.* 1996; 51:212–7.

57. Fleiss JL. Significance tests have a role in epidemiologic research: reaction. *Am J Pub Health.* 1987; 76:559–60.

58. Pocock SJ, Hughes MD. Estimation issues in clinical trials and overviews. *Stat Med.* 1990; 9:657–71.

59. Kupper LL, Hafner KB. How appropriate are popular sample size formulas? *Am Stat.* 1989; 43:101–5.

60. Cohen J. *Statistical Power Analysis for the Behavioral Sciences.* 2nd ed. Hillsdale, NJ: L Erlbaum Associates; 1988.

61. Moussa MAA. Exact conditional and predictive power in planning clinical trials. *Controlled Clin Trials.* 1989; 10:376–85.

62. Altman DG. Size of clinical trials. *Br Med J.* 1983; 286:1842–3.

63. Browner WS, Newman TB. Are all significant P values created equal? *N Engl J Med.* 1987; 257:2459–63.

64. Schneiweiss F, Uthoff VA. Sample size and postmarketing surveillance. *Drug Info J.* 1985; 19:13–6.

65. Freiman JA, Chalmers TC, Smith H, et al. The importance of beta, the Type II error and sample size in the design and interpretation of the randomized control trial. *N Engl J Med.* 1978; 299:690–4.

66. Borenstein M, Cohen J. *Statistical Power Analysis: A Computer Program.* Hillsdale NJ: L Erlbaum Associates; 1988.

67. Czeizel AE, Dudas I. Prevention of the first occurrence of neural-tube defects by periconceptional vitamin supplementation. *N Engl J Med.* 1992; 327:1832–35.

68. Subcutaneous Sumatriptan Study Group. Treatment of migraine attacks with sumatriptan. *N Engl J Med.* 1991; 325:316–21.

69. Lavori PW, Louis TA, Bailar JC, et al. Designs for experiments-parallel comparisons of treatment. *N Engl J Med.* 1983; 309:1291–8.

70. Arkin CF, Wachtel MS. How many patients are necessary to assess test performance? *JAMA*. 1990; 263:275–8.

71. Lydick E, Yawn BP. Clinical interpretation of health-related quality of life data. In: Staquet MJ, Hays RD, Fayers PM, eds. *Quality of Life Assessment in Clinical Trials*. New York: Oxford University Press; 1998:299–314.

72. Anderson RB. What does it mean?: anchoring psychosocial quality of life scale score changes with reference to concurrent changes in reported symptom distress. *Drug Info J*. 1999; 33:445–53.

73. Sackett DL. How to read clinical journals: I. Why to read them and how to start reading them critically. *CMA J*. 1981; 124:555–8.

74. Walker AM. Reporting the results of epidemiologic studies. *Am J Pub Health*. 1986; 76:556–8.

75. Savitz D. Comments about statistical testing and confidence intervals. *Am J Pub Health*. 1987; 77:237–8.

76. Poole C. Beyond the confidence interval. *Am J Pub Health*. 1987; 77:195–9.

77. DeRuoen TA. Comments about statistical testing and confidence intervals. *Am J Pub Health*. 1987; 77:237.

78. Lachenbrach PA, Clark VA, Cumberland WG, et al. Comments about statistical testing and confidence intervals. *Am J Pub Health*. 1987; 77:237.

79. Fleiss JL. Significance tests have a role in epidemiologic research: reaction. *Am J Pub Health*. 1987; 76:559–60.

# Discussion and Conclusions

---□---

➤ ☐22. Is a strong causal relationship established between the clinical outcome measured and the administration of the investigational drug?

➤ ☐23. Are the study results clinically important and generalizable to patients treated in the typical clinical practice setting?

---□---

This chapter focuses on how to review the discussion and conclusions section of an article about a clinical drug trial. Two important issues are addressed. The first is whether the investigator established a strong causal relationship between the clinical outcome measured and the investigational drug (Question 22). The second is the extent to which the results are generalized for use in a typical practice (Question 23).

Usually, the final part of any article, after the results, is the discussion and conclusions section. Journal editors vary in policies regarding how the final section is organized: some require that the discussion and conclusions sections be separate, while others suggest that the sections be combined. Unfortunately, a lengthy and comprehensive discussion section would be unusual in most publications because of space limitations. Thus, investigators are often limited in their discussion of results.

A separate discussion section generally involves the investigator's interpretation of the study results. The conclusions section, if it exists, follows the discussion and is usually expressed as a short summary of the study's purpose and results. Along with the abstract and title, these sections are the parts of the article most often read (especially a short conclusions section) to get a quick understanding of the trial.

These sections either separately or combined focus on how the study results answer the research questions described in the trial objectives or research hypotheses. Investigators should discuss how the objective was achieved or not achieved and explain possible inconsistencies or limitations of the trial methodology. New and important results should be emphasized and linked with previous research or with current knowledge. Recommendations regarding follow-up research to confirm the results can be provided, especially if contradictions are reported. The investigators should discuss the implications of reported results that contradict other research on the same drug treatment. Although results inconsistent with previous research can lead to new scientific insight, they may also be due to

- poor research design,

- differences in methodology or patient population used, or

- a biased interpretation by the investigators.

Most importantly, investigators should describe their conclusions clearly and base them on quantitative evidence.[1–3]

One primary purpose of the discussion and conclusions section is for the investigators to establish whether the investigational drug was effective and safe. In scientific terms, this task means establishing the internal validity of the findings. While no consistent procedure is routinely followed to establish efficacy and safety, the discussion should include a description of the causal relationship between the investigational drug and the observed clinical outcomes. In addition, a description of the method used to assess the relationship and to eliminate other potential causative factors should be included.[4–9]

After the results of the clinical drug trial are reported, the investigators should indicate how they can be applied to patients in everyday practice. This assessment focuses on the external validity or applicability of the reported results and is sometimes referred to as extrapolation, estimation, or induction. Extrapolation of the reported results is probably the most difficult task in scientific literature evaluation and involves making inferences beyond the results of the clinical drug trial. The inferences are often needed because of the constraints placed on the trial design to ensure that the study followed the appropriate scientific guidelines.[4–9]

Despite the difficulty associated with assessing the applicability of the reported results, extrapolation is necessary if the investigational drug is going to be used properly. Unwillingness to extrapolate limits the results to patients similar to those in the trial and unnecessarily restricts the potential value of the investigational drug. Any recommendations for use of a drug in clinical settings should be based on solid evidence that the benefits of therapy outweigh potential risks and preferably on the demonstration of the cost effectiveness of therapy. The importance of the findings to the clinical practice setting should be discussed and the implications for future research, but overly enthusiastic extrapolation should be avoided.[4-9]

## ☑ 22. Is a strong causal relationship established between the clinical outcome measured and the administration of the investigational drug?

The definition of causality is based on the science of philosophy and refers to a specific set (or locus) of events that takes place during a specified time frame (past, present, or future). Causality is determined either retrospectively or prospectively. The retrospective approach identifies an effect that has already occurred, followed by an assessment of its possible causes.[10-16]

The prospective method involves a prediction that a significant number of patients exposed to the investigational drug will respond in a predetermined manner. Case-control studies are often designed to address retrospective causal propositions, whereas cohort studies or clinical drug trials are most effective for developing prospective causal explanations.[10-16]

Causation in a clinical drug trial refers to the events that begin with the administration of the investigational drug and end with a change in a clinical outcome measure. The trial should demonstrate a direct linkage between the investigational drug administration and those outcome measures. The implication would be that the investigational drug altered the disease, resulting in improved outcomes. An example would be the investigator's attempt to show that the administration of a new anticonvulsant drug resulted in the elimination of partial seizures in patients undergoing an outpatient surgical procedure.

In assessing causality, the investigator should consider four possible explanations (Figure 9-1).[17-19] The true causal relationship (A) can be stated simply as follows: "if the investigational drug is administered, the clinical outcome will occur." However, alternative explanations must be addressed and refuted before this relationship is accepted. One is that a relationship exists between the investigational drug and the clinical outcome but in the opposite direction: the clinical outcome came before the drug was administered and may have actually created the need for the drug (B). This relationship should not occur in a properly designed clinical drug trial because the order in which the drug is administered and the clinical outcome is observed is carefully controlled.

Another explanation is that no true relationship occurs between the administration of the investigational drug and the clinical outcome, and the association is due to a chance occurrence (C). The probability of this explanation occurring should be minimized with significance tests (*see* Chapter 8).

The last explanation is that the association observed between the investigational and control drug is actually due to a third factor (D). This last explanation is called confounding and is the most complex and difficult factor to control.

**Figure 9-1** Four Types of Explanations

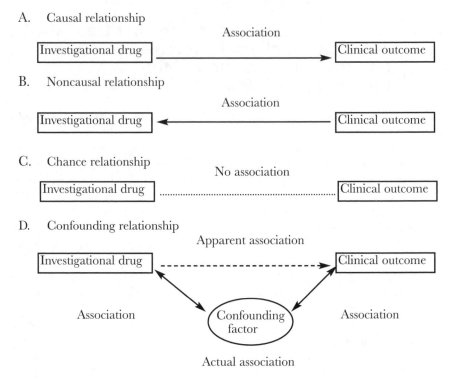

A. Causal relationship

B. Noncausal relationship

C. Chance relationship

D. Confounding relationship

## Confounding

Confounding is the general term for the effect of a third variable on the relationship between the administration of the investigational drug and the occurrence of the clinical outcome.[4,11,14,16,17,19–23] Confounding factors are those related to both the clinical outcome and drug administration and serve as the connecting link in the drug–effect relationship. An example would be the possibility that age would be a confounding factor in the use of hypnotic drugs. That is, older patients may respond more intensely to the investigational hypnotic drug than younger patients.

The impact of confounding may be addressed either in the design of the clinical drug trial or the data analysis. Design features include narrowing the type of patients included and stratified random assignment. Analytic procedures include the use of subgroup analysis or multivariate tests such as two-way ANOVA. The intent of these approaches is to separate the effects on the clinical outcome due to the confounding factor from the effects attributed to the investigational drug.

Causal relationships are much easier to establish in randomized control trials than in case-control or retrospective studies. Nevertheless, other criteria than the study design should be considered in assessing the strength of a causal relationship.

## Causality Criteria

The strength of a causal relationship should be evaluated directly or indirectly through the use of widely accepted criteria for assessing causality (Table 9-1).[4,24-26] Because most criteria are not systematically addressed by investigators in the discussion or conclusion sections, the reader must determine whether sufficient evidence is provided to establish a causal relationship. In addition, other sections may include important evidence that support causation. Meeting all criteria described in Table 9-1 would not unequivocally establish that the investigational drug caused the clinical outcomes, particularly if the trial design has flaws such as nonrandom assignment of patients, lack of double-blind techniques, or poor measures. Nevertheless, the probability of a strong causal relationship existing between the investigational drug and the clinical outcomes increases as the number of criteria met increases.

**Table 9-1** Criteria for Establishing Causality in Clinical Drug Trials[4,24-26]

| Criterion | Description |
|---|---|
| **Temporal relationship** | The clinical outcome should clearly occur after (not before) the investigational drug is administered to the patient. |
| **Strength** | The incidence of the clinical outcome reported in the experimental group should be higher than the incidence reported in the control group. |
| **Consistency** | The clinical outcomes reported in the clinical drug trial have been reported in other trials with the same investigational drug or with other drugs within the same class. |
| **Biological plausibility** | The relationship is biologically probable based on the current understanding of the investigational drug and the disease under treatment. |
| **Specificity** | The clinical outcome has a high probability of occurring when the investigational drug is given and is likely to be absent when the drug is not present. |
| **Dose-response effect** | The severity or magnitude of the clinical outcome increases with increasing doses or duration of the investigational drug. |

### *Temporal relationship*

The primary objective in establishing a temporal relationship is to ensure that the observed clinical outcomes occurred after (not before) the investigational drug was administered. This objective is often difficult to establish because the clinical outcomes may be due to many factors, especially the natural course of the disease. Theoretically, a randomized controlled trial should be effective in establishing a temporal relationship through the use of control groups containing similar patients (*see* Chapter 4). Because case-control or cohort studies do not routinely possess similar characteristics as a randomized control trial, a temporal relationship is more difficult to establish. Establishment of a temporal relationship in a randomized control trial is not guaranteed. Protocol deviations such as treating patients with a diagnosis lacking the expected outcome, including patients with concomitant diseases, patient noncompliance, concurrent use of interacting drugs, and variations in the data collection procedures can make establishing the temporal relationship more difficult.[16,24,26]

### Strength

The stronger the association between the administration of the investigational drug and the presence of the clinical outcome, the more likely it is that a causal relationship occurred.[24-29] The strength of a causal relationship is determined by the relative frequency of the expected clinical outcome in the experimental group compared to the control group. The strength is sometimes expressed as the relative risk, defined by the following formula and described extensively in Chapter 8, Question 20:

$$\text{relative risk} = \frac{\text{incidence of clinical outcome in experimental group}}{\text{incidence of clinical outcome in control group}}$$

No consistent guidelines exist regarding the desirable strength of the association necessary to establish a causal relationship. However, some journal editors and scientific organizations suggest that the relative risk (or possibility that the investigational drug caused the clinical outcome) should be equal to at least three times the incidence of the outcome in the control before causality can be established.[27]

Like temporal relationships, the strength of a causal relationship is established most easily in randomized controlled trials. Nonrandomized clinical drug trials are less likely to accurately estimate the strength of the relationship because there is less information about the similarity of the experimental and control patients. Even randomization does not ensure accurate estimation of the causal relationship's strength. Differences between the experimental and control group could be distorted in clinical drug trials that have only a few patients.[24-26,28,29]

### Consistency

Consistency is based on the expected reproducibility of the causal relationship.[1,2,24,26] Causality should be expected to occur across a wide range of patients in different settings. While reproducibility can sometimes be established in the same trial if patients are reexposed to the investigational drug, the usual method for establishing consistency is through the examination of previous research. Consistency means that different trials resulted in the same association, although the trial may have employed different designs conducted on different samples sometimes located in different countries.

If an association between an investigational drug and a clinical outcome is demonstrated repeatedly through various trials that utilize different samples and different study techniques, the probability of causation is increased. Consistency among poorly designed trials is helpful, although limited, because of the individual study weaknesses in methodology.[1,2,24,26]

The investigator's attempt to establish the consistency of the causal relationship is usually shown in the literature review at the beginning of the article, as well as in the discussion section. The review should include references to similar trials of the investigational drug. Inconsistent trial results suggest poor causality and should be explained. Information about drugs from the same class is often used to establish consistency because little information is usually available about an investigational drug.[1,2,24,26]

### Biologic plausibility

Biologic plausibility refers to the observed association being biologically understandable on the basis of current knowledge.[1,2,24,26] This criterion is sometimes referred to as the "coherence of the association." A causal relationship between the investigational drug and the expected clinical outcome must make biological sense based on the drug's mechanism of action, its pharmacokinetic and pharmacodynamic profile, and the underlying pathological mechanism of the disease. This information is initially accumulated in the preclinical research for a new drug and better established in phase I and II trials. It is later refined in phase III and IV clinical research.[1,2,24,26]

To establish the biological plausibility of the causal relationship, the investigators should provide background information from prior research and existing clinical practice about the expected and unexpected effects of the investigational drug. This information is usually provided in the literature review, with additional references in the discussion section. Because almost any potential causal relationship can be made to sound biologically plausible, the investigators need to provide sufficient background information to justify their assertions. Information from drugs of the same class may be used in situations where the newness of the investigational drug restricts the availability of similar information.[1,2,24,26]

## *Specificity*

Specificity is determined by the distinctness of the causal relationship and measures the degree in which administration of the investigational drug produces a specific outcome. The expected clinical outcome should appear after the investigational drug is administered, but not if the drug was not present. If a variable clinical response occurs, the relationship is less likely to be causal. In a clinical drug trial, specificity is more likely to occur when the clinical outcome is clearly described and narrowly defined. Specificity is difficult to establish in a clinical research trial because most clinical outcomes have multiple causes besides the investigational drug. In addition, investigational drugs rarely cause the expected clinical outcomes in all patients.[5,24,26,30]

Specificity is justified by the investigator in many sections of the article, particularly the description of the methodology and the results. It is often measured by the probability that a specific association between the investigational drug and the clinical outcome occurs. This probability results from a comparison of the experimental and control groups. A higher incidence of the clinical outcome in the experimental group would suggest a specific relationship, especially if it is statistically significant and derived from a randomized controlled trial with a minimal amount of patient withdrawal. This probability is often enhanced through subgroup analysis, which may further clarify the conditions in which the association occurs.[5,24,26,30]

## *Dose–response effect*

The dose–response effect consists of an expected change in the clinical outcomes when the dose or duration of the investigational drug is changed.[24,26] The consideration of the dose–response relationship is similar to that of strength. In a causal relationship, increasing the dose of the investigational drug should result in a corresponding change in the clinical outcome. The change should always be in one direction (either an increase or decrease in the effect) and should be as close to linear as possible.[24,26]

In clinical drug trials, dose–response relationships are initially established early in the research about the investigational drug, usually in preclinical and phase I and II trials. It is later refined in phase III and IV studies. Because of the methodological and analytical complexities of a clinical drug trial involving different doses of the investigational drug, the dose–response relationship is infrequently assessed in a single trial. Thus, substantial prior evidence about this relationship should be presented in the literature review.[24,26]

However, further justification can be established through the design of the clinical drug trial and the subsequent results. A dose–response effect would be difficult to assess in those conditions in which a quantitative assessment of the patient response is not possible. An example may be the evaluation of an antiinfective drug in which the clinical outcome is measured by the nominal scale of presence or absence of symptoms. No range of response would be possible with this type of scale.[24,26]

# ☑ 23. Are the study results clinically important and generalizable to patients treated in the typical clinical practice setting?

Assessing the value of the results of a clinical drug trial is complex and is influenced by many groups' perspective. These groups include the drug sponsor, the Food and Drug Administration (FDA), the patient, the healthcare practitioner, healthcare institutions and managed care organizations, consumer groups, and the investment community. From a financial perspective, the trial results need to be sufficient to get the drug approved, marketed, and used clinically.[9,31,32]

From a regulatory perspective, the results must demonstrate that the drug is safe enough to be used clinically and efficacious enough to add benefit for patients suffering from the disease. Organizations involved in healthcare delivery (e.g., hospitals and managed care organizations) are interested in the cost effectiveness of the drug compared to existing treatment. While all of these perspectives are important, the most important assessment should come from the healthcare practitioner and the patient.[9,31,32]

## Clinical Significance

The assessment of the value of the results of a clinical drug trial to patients and healthcare practitioners depends on several factors. A primary factor is the establishment that the investigational drug is strongly associated with the clinical outcomes measured. Once causality (internal validity) has been verified, the magnitude of the investigational drug's effect on the clinical outcome compared to the control treatment must be assessed.[12,27,33–42]

The establishment of a strong causal relationship that results in a large comparative difference is an important condition for establishing the clinical significance of the results. However, other factors are also needed for the results to be considered clinically important. These include the relative magnitude of the difference and the potential for the results changing the way patients suffering from the disease are treated (*see* Table 8-8, Chapter 8).

The healthcare practitioner usually subjectively determines these factors based on the information provided in the study and the investigator's beliefs about the importance of the results. Although this approach is individualized and somewhat arbitrary, efforts have been undertaken to make it more systematic through the applications of evidence-based practice. Table 9-2 illustrates some factors used by the healthcare practitioner to assess clinical significance. These factors focus on the study methodology, the plan used to analyze the data, and the investigator's interpretation of the study results.[12,27,33–42]

**Table 9-2**  Factors Used to Assess the Clinical Significance of the Results of Clinical Drug Trials

| Factors | Description |
| --- | --- |
| Comparison of strategies | The comparison should be between the investigational drug and the most likely alternative treatment available for the patient suffering from the disease. Clinical drug trials that use placebo controls are less valuable. |
| Investigator bias | Well-designed clinical drug trials minimize the extent of investigator bias. However, bias can still occur in the interpretation of the results. Of particular concern are investigators who emphasize results from analysis of the secondary study objectives, from only particular outcome measures, or from selective subgroup analyses. |
| Presentation of information | The results of the clinical drug trial should be summarized in easy-to-understand formats by which the probability of the clinical outcome occurring after administration of the investigation is presented. Separate probabilities for each outcome should be displayed. |
| Selection of clinical outcomes to measure | The clinical drug trial should include outcomes that matter to the patient and the healthcare practitioner. Generally these include meaningful clinical outcomes such as mortality, cure of disease, and drug safety. Quality of life measures are also important. |
| Study methodology and data quality | Clinical drug trials that include appropriate patient selection and enrollment procedures, randomized controls, double-blind observations, and reliable, appropriate, and valid measures are likely to produce high quality data. Poor quality data are less likely to be used to change clinical practice. |

## Generalizability

Once the results are considered clinically significant, the healthcare practitioner needs to know whether the findings are generalizable to patients in practice.[30,36–41,43–46] The assessment involves estimating the external validity of the results. If study conditions are not similar to those routinely encountered in clinical situations, the results may not be applicable to patient care. The investigator can aid in this assessment by discussing the results in relation to findings from previous studies and research.

Assessing the generalizability of the trial results usually involves comparing the characteristics of the trial with similar characteristics likely to be present in everyday practice. Some characteristics are related to the patient (age, gender, race, or medical condition), the medical setting (ambulatory or inpatient), or the drug regimen (dose forms or schedules) used.[30,36-41,43-46]

Other characteristics are related to the methodology used, such as the potential biases in the subject selection procedure or poor measures used for assessing the efficacy and safety of the clinical drug trial. Even if few errors are made in extrapolation, healthcare practitioners should be cautious about making changes based on a single trial. Results need to be repeated and experience gained in broader populations before the true efficacy and safety of the investigational drug are established.[30,36-41,43-46]

# References

1. Hamilton CW. How to write and publish scientific papers: scribing information for pharmacists. *Am J Hosp Pharm.* 1992; 49:2477–84.

2. Walker AM. Reporting the results of epidemiologic studies. *Am J Pub Health.* 1986; 76:556–8.

3. Nahata MC. Publishing by pharmacists. *Drug Intell Clin Pharm.* 1989; 23:809–10.

4. Greenland S. Randomization, statistics and causal inference. *Epidemiology.* 1990; 1:421–9.

5. Koch GG, Sollecito WA. Statistical considerations in the design, analysis and interpretation of comparative clinical studies. *Drug Info J.* 1984; 18:131–51.

6. O'Brien PC, Shampo MA. Statistics for clinicians: epilogue. *Mayo Clinic Proc.* 1981; 56:755–6.

7. Riegelman RK, Hirsch RP. *Studying a Study and Testing a Test: How to Read the Medical Literature.* 2nd ed. Boston: Little Brown; 1989.

8. Moses LE. Statistical concepts fundamental to investigations. In: Bailar JC, Mosteller F, eds. *Medical Use of Statistics.* Boston: NEJM Books; 1992:5–25.

9. Lasagna L. Balancing risks versus benefits in drug therapy decisions. *Clin Ther.* 1998; 20:C72–C79.

10. Elwood MJ. *Critical Appraisal of Epidemiological Studies and Clinical Trials.* New York: Oxford University Press; 1998:218–44.

11. Morton RF, Hebel JR, McCarter RJ. *A Study Guide to Epidemiology and Biostatistics.* 4th ed. Gaithersburg MD: Aspen; 1996.

12. Ahbolm A; *Biostatistics for Epidemiologists.* Ann Arbor: Lewis Publishers; 1993.

13. Kramer MS, Lane DA. Causal propositions in clinical research and practice. *J Clin Epidemiol.* 1992; 45:639–49.

14. Kirby D. Adverse drug events in clinical trials. In: Solgliero-Gilbert G, ed. *Drug Safety Assessment in Clinical Trials.* 3rd ed. New York: Marcel Dekker; 1993:25–38.

15. Hutchinson TA, Lane DA. Standardized methods of causality assessment for suspected adverse drug reactions. *J Chron Dis.* 1986; 39:857–60.

16. Gray-Donald K, Kramer MK. Causality inference in observational vs experimental studies. *J Epidemiol.* 1988; 127:885–93.

17. Elwood MJ. *Critical Appraisal of Epidemiological Studies and Clinical Trials.* New York: Oxford University Press; 1998:116–60.

18. Maclure M. Multivariate refutation of etiological hypotheses in nonexperimental epidemiology. *Int J Epidemiol.* 1990; 19:782–7.

19. Gehlbach SH. *Interpreting the Medical Literature: A Clinician's Guide: Practical Epidemiology for Clinicians.* 2nd ed. New York: Macmillan; 1988:70–4.

20. Savitz D. Comments about statistical testing and confidence intervals. *Am J Pub Health.* 1987; 77:237–8.

21. Oxman AD, Guyatt GH. A consumer's guide to subgroup analysis. *Ann Intern Med.* 1992; 116:76–84.

22. Haunsperger DB, Saari DG. The lack of consistency for statistical decision procedures. *Am Stat.* 1991; 45:252–5.

23. O'Brien PC, Shampo MA. Statistics for clinicians: 6. Comparing two samples (the two-sample t test). *Mayo Clinic Proc.* 1981; 56:393–4.

24. Trout KS. How to read clinical journals: IV. To determine etiology or causation. *CMA J.* 1981; 124:985–90.

25. Johnson JM. Reasonable possibility: causality and postmarketing surveillance. *Drug Info J.* 1992; 26:553–8.

26. Hill AB. *Principles of Medical Statistics.* 9th ed. New York: Oxford University Press; 1971:309–27.

27. Gibaldi M. Do calcium antagonists pose a risk to patients with hypertension. *Pharmaceutical News.* 1996; 3:8–12.

28. Morton RF, Hebel JR, McCarter RJ. *A Study Guide to Epidemiology and Biostatistics.* 3rd ed. Rockville MD: Aspen; 1990:35–46.

29. Koch GG, Hartzema AG. Basic statistical methods in pharmacoepidemiologic study designs. In: Hartzema AG, Porta MS, Tilson HH, eds. *Pharmacoepidemiology: An Introduction.* Cincinnati, OH: Harvey Whitney Books, 1990:142–75.

30. Oye RK, Shapiro MF. Reporting results from chemotherapy trials: does response make a difference in patient survival? *JAMA.* 1984; 252:2722–5.

31. Brown GB. The changing audience for clinical trials. *Drug Info J.* 1995; 29:591–8.

32. Pathek DS, Escovitz A. Assuring the safe use of medications: the drug approval process and improving treatment decisions. *Clin Ther.* 1998; 20:C1–C4.

33. Rosenberg WM, Sackett DL. On the need for evidence-based medicine. *Therapie.* 1996; 51:212–7.

34. Committee on Clinical Practice Guidelines, Institute of Medicine; *Guidelines for Clinical Practice.* Washington DC: National Academy Press; 1992.

35. Pearson KC. Role of evidence-based medicine and clinical practice guidelines in treatment decisions. *Clin Ther.* 1998; 20:C80–C85.

36. Richardson WS, Detsky AS. User's guide to the medical literature: VII. How to use a clinical decision model. A. Are the results of the study valid? *JAMA.* 1995; 273:1610–3.

37. Richardson WS, Detsky AS. User's guide to the medical literature: VII. How to use a clinical decision model. B. What are the results and will they help me in caring for my patients? *JAMA.* 1995; 273:1292–5.

38. Naylor DC, Chen E, Strauss B. Measured enthusiasm: does the method of reporting trial results alter perceptions of therapeutic effectiveness? *Ann Intern Med.* 1992; 117:916–21.

39. Davies HTO, Crombie IK. Outcomes from observational studies: understanding causal ambiguity. *Drug Info J.* 1999; 33:153–8.

40. Lucas BD, Hillerman DE. Media sensationalism of clinical trials: freedom of information or potential for causing patient harm? *Ann Pharmacother.* 1995; 29:629–31.

41. Berzon RA. Understanding and using health-related quality of life instruments within clinical research studies. In: Staquet MJ, Hays RD, Fayers PM, eds. *Quality of Life Assessment in Clinical Trials.* New York: Oxford University Press; 1998:3–15.

42. DeMets D. Distinction between fraud, bias, errors, misunderstanding, and incompetence. *Controlled Clin Trials.* 1997; 18:637–50.

43. Feinstein AR. Clinical biostatistics I: a new name--and some other changes of the guard. *Clin Pharmacol Ther.* 1970; 11:135–48.

44. Bailar JC. Some uses of statistical thinking. In: Bailar JC, Mosteller F, eds. *Medical Use of Statistics.* Boston: NEJM Books; 1992:27–44.

45. O'Connell JB, Mason JW. The applicability of results of streamlined trials to clinical practice: the myocarditis treatment trial. *Stat Med.* 1990; 9:193–7.

46. Murphy EA. Public and private hypotheses. *J Clin Epidemiol.* 1989; 42:79–84.

# INDEX

In this index, page numbers in italics designate figures; page numbers followed by "t" designate tables. *See also* cross-references designate related topics or more detailed topic breakdowns.

# D E F

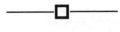